Superfoods Explained

A Guide To Health & Nutrition

What are superfoods, healthy eating, superfoods list, diet, weight loss, recipes, shopping list, tips, and more!

By Cynthia Cherry

Copyrights and Trademarks

Disclaimer and Legal Notice

Foreword

Are superfoods a nutritional magic bullet? No. The main reason to take a nutritionally dense cross section of foods and set them apart under the "super" label is this: in all our modernity, we've forgotten how to eat.

Let me single out just one of my pet nutritional peeves to try to elucidate my point. It's been just about 45 years since high-fructose corn syrup was introduced into the American diet as a low cost sweetener.

Since that time, obesity rates have shot up in the United States to the now alarming levels. In 1970, only about 15% of Americans were clinically obese. Now, it's more than a third of the total adult population. That's roughly 78.7 million people.

A great deal of the blame for that falls squarely on high-fructose corn syrup, a staple in processed foods. This stuff is everywhere: soda, cereal, fruit juice, bread, mayonnaise, yogurt, peanut butter. I have to dig through the ketchup bottles at the store to find one that's labeled "no high fructose corn syrup!"

Over-consumption of sugar can be just as damaging in a healthy diet, but consider this alarming fact. High-fructose corn syrup has been linked to colony collapse disorder among honeybees. Feeding this replacement food to the bees has weakened their natural immunity and made them more susceptible to pesticides, so they are dying off in huge numbers.

No matter how many defenders come forward to insist high fructose corn syrup is safe, it is a highly processed substance that is in no way natural. If it can change the metabolism of a honey bee, it certainly has the ability to change ours as well. Given the rising obesity rates, it would appear to have done that very thing.

Why are we relying on heavily processed and now genetically modified foods when we have so many options for nutritionally dense "real" foods from which to choose? Why have we so polluted our food supply that we have to worry about contamination from pesticides and fertilizers? Why do we support a food industry that makes such contaminated food available at cheap prices while organic products are more expensive?

If you want to be a food "super" hero, the reason you are reading this book is not to find a magic bullet, but to find your way back to real food. I will admit that I am an advocate of a primarily plant-based diet, but your first goal in eating healthy is to re-discover simple, affordable foods that are packed with healthy compounds and build your new diet around those items.

Acknowledgments

I would like to express my gratitude towards my friends and colleagues for their kind co-operation and encouragement which helped me in completion of this book.

I would like to express my special gratitude and thanks to my loving husband for his patience, understanding, and support.

My thanks and appreciations also go to my colleagues and people who have willingly helped me out with their abilities.

Additional thanks to my family, whose love and my concern for their wellbeing inspired me to write this book.

Table of Contents

Table of Contents

Table of Contents

Table of Contents

Chapter 1 - What Are Superfoods?

"Super" foods aren't "super-sized" like the not-so-healthy meals from a certain fast food chain. Instead, these are foods that deliver the greatest nutritional value to your body to maximize your health and to protect you against the effects of disease and aging.

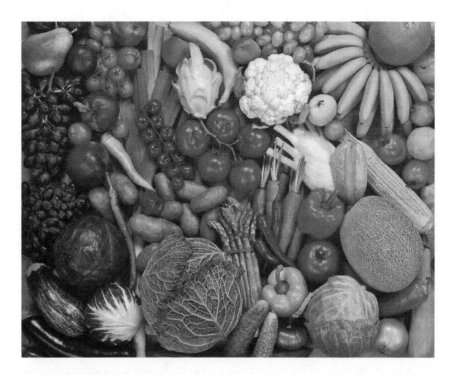

Using Food As Medicine

The idea of using food as medicine is fundamental to all the world's healing traditions, especially those in China, India, and Greece. Going even farther back to our hunter-gatherer ancestors, learning about medicinal herbs and beneficial plants was simply an aspect of survival that in time became refined to actual "prescribed" remedies.

Now the traditional connection between food and medicine is being "validated" by modern science for what it really is, a practical and natural way to manage health and to *prevent* illness rather than treat it after the fact. Rather than reacting after the fact, eating to maximize health is proactive, coast effective, and life enhancing.

Far from being a "discovery," superfoods and sound dietary practices are being "re-discovered" in a time when far more people are eating "food-like" substances rather than real food and paying the price with poor health and high medical bills.

What Are Blue Zones?

As "proof of concept," let's look at the idea of the "Blue Zones." This term grew out of the work of Gianni Pes and Michel Poulain who demographically proved that the Nuoro province of Sardinia was home to the world's highest population of male centenarians.

When the researchers become more focused on the regions with the greatest longevity, they drew concentric blue circles on their maps. As a kind of shorthand, the men began to refer to the areas inside the circles as "Blue Zones," a term now used to describe areas of the world where people live significantly longer lives, often in excess of 100 years. These regions include:

- Okinawa (Japan)
- Sardinia (Italy)
- Nicoya (Costa Rica)
- Icaria (Greece)
- Seventh-Day Adventist communities in Loma Linda, California

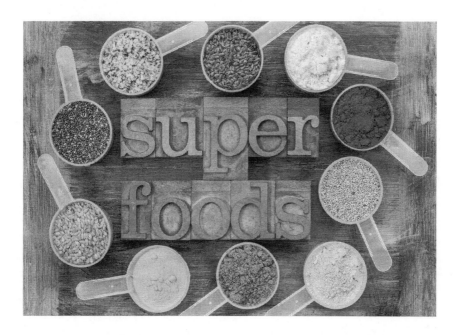

But it's not just a matter of living longer, people inside the Blue Zones are also living better. In Icaria, Greece for instance, residents enjoy a 20% lower cancer rate, 50% less heart disease, and almost no dementia.

In trying to understand exactly what makes Blue Zones unique, six lifestyle characteristics stand out according to Dan Buettner, author of *The Blue Zones: 9 Lessons for Living Longer From the People Who've Lived the Longest*:

- An emphasis on family above all other concerns.
- Little to no use of tobacco.
- Semi-vegetarianism. (Sardinia is the exception.)
- Common consumption of legumes.
- A constant level of moderate physical activity.
- Social engagement with friends and as part of the community.

Beyond the benefits clearly derived from family and social engagement, these people are consuming diets that emphasize nutrient-dense "super" foods.

Superfoods and Nutrient Density

Simply put, foods that are nutrient dense have more essential nutrients by volume and fewer calories. Say, for instance, that you're hungry after you've already had lunch and start looking for a snack about the middle of the afternoon. Your choices are an apple or a glazed donut.

Both are about the same size. The donut has approximately 200 calories and 1 gram of fiber. It tastes good and if there are more in the box, you may eat a second or a third before you're full because a single donut won't fill you up.

The apple has 80 calories and is packed with vitamins, phytochemicals, and 3.6-4.6 grams of fiber. Eat the apple and it will satisfy you until supper because its density equals that of three glazed donuts. Low calorie foods with high nutrient density are clearly good for weight loss and maintenance, and most of them also qualify as "superfoods" for a host of other reasons.

Nutrient-Dense Superfoods

You'll see many items on short and long lists of superfoods. As a general rule of thumb, when you're shopping, stay on the edges of the store where you'll find produce, lean meats, and low fat dairy items. That's superfood territory.

The middle regions of the grocery store are the land of processed, packaged foods that may or may not be good for you, a determination you can't make without a PhD in label reading. Even then, there's no guarantee of full disclosure in regard to ingredients.

But once you learn which foods you like that are also nutrient dense superfoods, your choices become much simpler and the guess work is eliminated.

The bottom line is this. What you eat affects your health. You can good make choices that maximize nutrition. In doing so you support weight loss and the chance for a longer life free of cardiovascular disease, cancer, diabetes, and cognitive impairment from aging. Let's single out cancer to further explore these assertions.

Food and Cancer

According to the American Cancer Society and the American Institute for Cancer Research, eating right, exercising more, and not smoking can eliminate more than 50 percent of cancers. By making better lifestyle choices, more than half of the cancer diagnoses made every year can just go away!

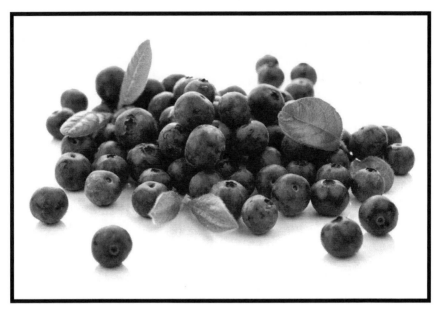

This staggering effect comes from a diet that emphasizes fruits, vegetables, and healthy meat like fish. These foods introduce essential fiber while lowering inflammation in the body. They contain antioxidants and nutrients that eliminate the activity of free radicals and the tissue damage they cause.

Fruits and vegetables linked to low cancer rates include (but are not limited to): carrots, sweet potatoes, spinach, kale, papaya, tomatoes, cauliflower, cabbage, cress, bok choy, broccoli, blueberries, blackberries, and garlic.

Various population studies point to the importance of raising levels of Vitamins A, B, C, E, D, and certain types of carotenoids to lower the risk of cancer – elements delivered by these fruits and vegetables.

Clearly, understanding the specific nutritional mechanism associated with plant-based foods is essential in making your selections. That information does not stop at vitamins and minerals, however. Biologically active compounds called phytonutrients are also important for their role in protecting the body against many forms of disease, not just cancer.

Obesity And Weight Loss Obsession

Although many people are unwilling to admit it, obesity is a disease and one that has reached epidemic levels in the United States. Since the 1970s, obesity rates for adults and children have more than doubled, giving birth to a burgeoning diet industry.

Retail bookshelves are packed with books recommending this or that eating plan or describing surgeries that remove part of the intestines to reduce how much a person can consume.

Would someone really consider weight loss methods that drastic? Yes, amazingly they would. Some people are so resistant to eating a plant-based diet they'd rather opt for surgery or spend thousands of dollars on diet pills and medications to manage their illnesses – all stemming from obesity.

These choices are also driven by the medical and pharmaceutical industries whose job it is to convince people to undergo procedures or buy their products. Since there's no big money in broccoli, you can see where the advertising dollars are spent.

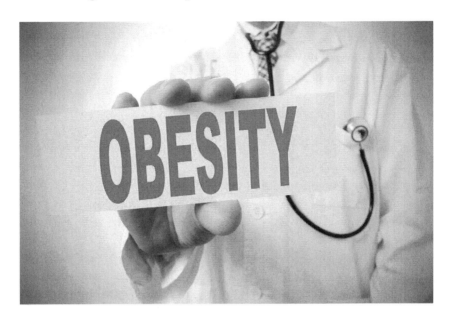

A change to a mostly plant-based diet, comprised primarily of the superfoods listed in this book, will actually allow you to eat as much as you like without concern for calories.

Your weight loss will happen because of the foods you are eating, not due to any extreme diet fads or calorie counting. Being thin does not necessarily mean that you are healthy. Eating a predominantly plant-based diet will ensure that you are healthy as well as the correct weight.

Superfoods vs Exercise

Most of us assume we'll grow old and die. Of course we all realize that we will die eventually, but the more likely truth is that you will grow old and live. Life expectancy is rising, which is a good thing, but it also means that disease and illness are almost certain to be a part of your future – unless you do something to change the odds. The quality of your life as you age should be of the utmost importance to you and something you actively work to improve on all levels.

While it is true that adding superfoods to your diet will return health benefits, exercise is equally important. People who live longer all incorporate physical activity into their lifestyle as a daily habit.

Exercise not only improves your physical well-being, it also boosts brain function regardless of age or fitness level and delivers a range of unexpected benefits:

- **Stress reduction.** Working out increases levels of norepinephrine, which moderates the brain's stress responses and relieves anxiety.

- **Feel good endorphins.** When we exercise, our bodies release endorphins, which make us feel happier, even euphoric. Exercise can alleviate depression and anxiety even if you're only breaking a sweat for 30 minutes 2 or 3 times a week. Short exercise sessions substituting endorphin release for drugs and alcohol are also helpful in treating addiction.

- **Improved self-confidence.** Regardless of size, weight, or gender, exercise has been proven to improve self-perception and with it feelings of self-worth.

- **Boost Vitamin D levels.** If you take your exercise outdoors (maybe doing something that's fun *and* healthy), you'll also benefit from soaking up Vitamin D from sunshine, a nutrient only found nutritionally in oily fish.

- **Stay mentally sharp.** To hold aging and mental deteriation at bay, working out enhances brain function, especially in the area of the hippocampus, the region of the brain that controls memory and learning. It's also been proven that cardiovascular exercise actually stimulates the growth of new brain cells.

- **Improve relaxation.** Exercising 5-6 hours before bedtime raises the body's core temperature. When it falls a few hours later, it serves as a signal that it's time for sleep. A moderate workout can be better for insomnia that a sleeping pill.

- **Jumpstart your brain.** If you're stuck at work and feeling uninspired and sleepy, get up and take a brisk walk around the block. The moderate exercise will wake you up and give your creative powers a boost for at least two hours.

While most of us have a hard time starting an exercise program, we enjoy the benefits once they become apparent in our lives. Superfoods can't do it all! Help them out with a moderate amount of exercise to bring yourself closer to your goals for long-term health and well-being.

Chapter 2 - The Super Fruits

Like vegetables, super fruits offer powerful protection against heart attack, stroke, cancer, type 2 diabetes, high blood pressure, bone loss, and weight gain. Fruits are naturally low fat and low sodium and they have zero cholesterol.

Fruits also give us access to under-consumed nutrients like dietary fiber, Vitamin C, folate, and potassium. Because most are naturally sweet, these are nature's best "treats," livening our diets with both flavor and color.

Apples

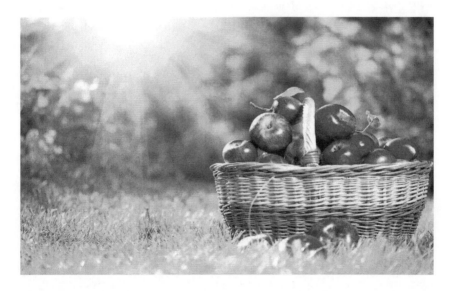

The old adage about "an apple a day" is true! A medium-sized apple is only 100 calories with no fat. The more apples you eat, the more you control your hunger with beneficial calories that ward off cancer, cardiovascular disease, diabetes, and asthma.

Apples are an excellent source of Vitamin C and they're full of antioxidants. These phytochemicals not only give the fruit its brilliant red hue, they combat damage caused by free radicals in our systems.

Free radicals aren't just associated with cancer, but also with inflammation, hardening of the arteries, and neurological disorders including Parkinson's and Alzheimer's.

The good news doesn't stop there. Any fruit with white flesh, like apples and pears, lowers our risk of stroke. Packed full of fiber, these fruits improve digestive function for better weight loss and higher immunological response.

Apricots

In an odd twist, the humble apricot, an often-neglected source of Vitamin A, is actually better in dried form. Full of beta-carotene, which brings down cholesterol levels, apricots are good to ward off heart disease and to protect the body from cancer. As an added benefit, they're also fantastic for eye health.

A couple of handfuls add up to 300 calories, so be mindful of your portions. Use dried apricots in homemade granola or in dishes like Moroccan tagine where they boost the flavor. Get creative. Go after the benefit of this common fruit without over doing it.

Avocado

People shy away from avocados because they contain the most fat of any fruit. All of the fat, however, is monosaturated, which guards against heart disease.

Avocados also have 30 % of the daily-recommended intake of fiber per cup, which is instrumental in lowering cholesterol levels.

You will know you have a ripe avocado in your hand if the skin gives under your fingers, but is still firm. If the consistency if mushy, the fruit is overly ripe. Don't try to go by the color of the skin, since there are hundreds of varieties.

Don't think guacamole is the only use for delicious avocados. Work them into salads or soups, or just eat them fresh sliced as a colorful addition to your dinner plate.

(If you want to keep your avocados from turning brown once sliced, add lemon or lime juice, which will slow the oxidation process.)

Bananas

With 3 grams of fiber per average banana, this common fruit is excellent for weight loss as a nutritious and sweet snack. At the same time, bananas contain impressive levels of Vitamin C, Vitamin B6, and carotenoids (which increase Vitamin A levels in the body.)

The potassium in bananas (420 mg of the daily recommended adult intake) helps keep electrolytes in balance and is good for proper function of the cells, tissues, and organs. Potassium is also believed to play a beneficial role in regulating blood pressure.

Blackberries, Blueberries, Strawberries

The brilliant purple that makes *blackberries* so beautiful is a signal of their high levels of anthocyanins, natural compounds that support memory function and anti-aging while guarding against cancer.

With more than half of the daily-recommended dosage of Vitamin C, the berries are fantastic for cardiovascular function, the immune system, and skin health. They have 6 grams of fiber to optimize digestion and are rich in anti-carcinogenic antioxidants called phenolic acids.

Eat blackberries fresh or frozen in everything from jam to wine! They are delicious when added to smoothies, and in pies, cobblers, and other desserts. Blackberries are in season from the end of the summer into the beginning of fall.

Blueberries are equally packed with antioxidants and are especially good for brain health, enhancing memory and increasing learning capacity in older individuals. The berries could reduce cognitive decline and actually fight the devastating effects of Alzheimer's and Parkinson's.

One cup contains 24% of the daily-recommended dose of Vitamin C and 14% of the suggested fiber intake for an adult. Studies indicate that eating a cup of blueberries per week will speed up the metabolism and lower blood pressure, again due to the presence of anthocyanins.

Blueberries lower blood sugar and fight depression. They are thought to inhibit the growth of breast cancer cells, to reduce the risk of coronary disease, and to lower LDL cholesterol.

The best season for fresh blueberries is May to October. Get as creative as you like with them in your recipes, but don't forget about just washing them and enjoying the berries a handful at a time.

Strawberries are rich in Vitamin C that actively repairs and builds the tissues while boosting immunity. Vitamin C improves eye health and even decreases the formation of wrinkles. The berries have also been linked to lower cholesterol levels.

A single cup of strawberries satisfies the daily Vitamin C requirement for men and women. They are high in manganese and have a good amount of fiber. At just 49 calories a serving, strawberries are wonderfully diet friendly, but be certain you don't have a strawberry allergy before digging in.

The best season for strawberries is April in Texas and Florida, May in the Deep South, and June in the Northern states.

Cantaloupe

Cantaloupe is a member of the gourd family. It has a sweet flavor and a juicy consistency perfect for taking the place of sugary desserts and snacks. A single cup has only 50 calories, but delivers 100% of the daily-recommended requirement for Vitamins A and C.

The Vitamin C fights off cancer, cardiovascular disease, cataracts, and the common cold, while Vitamin A prevents acne, clogged skin pores, and wrinkles. Its protective qualities may even extend to shielding the skin against the damaging effects of UV rays and ozone.

Since cantaloupe is 89% water and carries high levels of potassium, it's ideal for the hot summer months when dehydration can knock electrolyte levels out of balance.

Cantaloupe is available year round, but is freshest in June, July, and August. They may be kept at room temperature or refrigerated.

Cherries

Cherries are closely related to plums and peaches. There are sweet and sour varieties. Both average around 90 calories per cup and are full of protein, fiber, Vitamin C, and Vitamin A.

Like many richly hued fruits and vegetables, cherries are full of antioxidants called anthocyanins. Cherry juice is a great choice for an after-workout drink because it is a natural anti-inflammatory, aiding in muscle recovery with less accompanying pain.

These same anti-inflammatory properties may fight against arthritis, gout, diabetes, and cardiovascular disease. In laboratory studies, rats given cherry consumption exhibited lower blood levels of cholesterol and triglycerides.

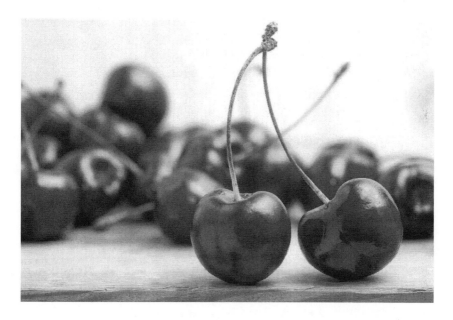

Cherries can also help fight the near epidemic level of sleep deprivation in our modern society. The fruit contains the hormone melatonin, which helps the body to correctly regulate its sleeping and waking cycles.

For people suffering from insomnia, additional melatonin is often all that's needed for a restful night of sleep without the use of potentially addictive medications. If you have chronic insomnia and need to pull out the big guns, eat

Montmorency tart cherries. They have six times more melatonin than any other variety.

Take advantage of cherries during the summer growing season. That's when you'll find fresh, plump, dark fruit at the peak of its nutritional effectiveness. Store cherries in the original packaging and do not wash them. This will prevent over-ripening and help the fruit to last for up to five days (longer if the stems are intact.)

Cranberries

Cranberries are packed with antioxidants, Vitamin C, and fiber. The berries have long been a folk remedy to ward off urinary tract infections and this is not just an old wives' tale.

Cranberries are anti-bacterial and anti-inflammatory, to the point that they lower the risk of heart disease, improve oral health, fight yeast infections, and prevent stomach ulcers. They may even stop the growth of cancer cells.

The optimal "dose" is one 10-ounce class per day. Stay away from cranberry juice "cocktails" and jellies full of sugar and opt for fresh juiced, dried, or frozen cranberries.

You can find fresh cranberries from September to December. They will keep up to 2 months in the refrigerator. They're great in sauces, relishes, cereals, and baked goods and it's near impossible to cook a Thanksgiving meal and not include cranberries on the table.

Grapes

Grapes come in all shades from red and purple to white. They are all considered berries and are bursting with powerful antioxidants including Vitamin C, Vitamin K, and beta-carotene to fight free radicals. One of the most intriguing phytonutrients found in grapes, however is resveratrol.

In recent years, resveratrol has made the headlines for its ability to lower LDL cholesterol, prevent damage to blood vessels, inhibit the growth of cancer cells, and even fight cognitive impairment.

Use grape seed oil, which is high in conjugated linoleic acid, to improve the quality of the skin and stop the enzymes that destroy elastin and cause wrinkles.

Grapes don't have a dramatic effect on blood sugar, so they are low on the glycemic index, but one cup does have 20 grams of sugar. That's the highest level for any fruit, so don't overdo it.

When buying, pick plumb grapes that are free of wrinkles. You want the ones that are fully ripe, but not starting to leak juice. That's a sign the bunch is about to spoil.

Since dark-skinned grapes have anthocyanins, which boost memory and improve motor function, they're a better nutritional choice over green grapes. Also, the darker the grape, the sweeter it will taste.

Grapes will keep for five days in a sealed plastic container. Wash the bunch when you get home from the store and dry it thoroughly.

Kiwi

The nutritionally dense kiwi promotes weight loss and helps to manage chronic digestive issues and asthma. Eating 2-3 kiwis per day can lower blood triglyceride levels by as much as 15 percent.

One medium kiwi offers an impressive list of the daily-recommended amounts of the following vitamins:

- 5% folate
- 117% Vitamin C
- 38% Vitamin K

How does the compare to other fruits? Eat a cup of sliced kiwi and you get 273% of the Vitamin C you need each day (along with 5 grams of fiber). A cup of oranges will only give you 160%.

Kiwi's list of minerals includes calcium, iron, magnesium, phosphorous, copper, and manganese. There is more potassium in one kiwi than in a sliced banana, with less sugar and fewer calories – only about 50 calories for one medium fruit and only 7 grams of sugar. That's even 3 times less than an apple!

Buy kiwi fruit that is fragrant, plump, and slightly firm to the touch. The skin is edible, and contains extra fiber, but most people prefer kiwi peeled.

Wash the fruit and gently rub the surface to remove the brown fuzz. If you don't want to bother slicing the kiwi, cut it in two and slice out the flesh with a spoon.

Lemons

The juice from a single lemon will give you one-third of the daily-recommended intake of Vitamin C (and just 12 calories) along with powerful flavonoids to:

- decrease the risk of heart attack
- reduce inflammation
- fight off pancreatic and stomach cancer.

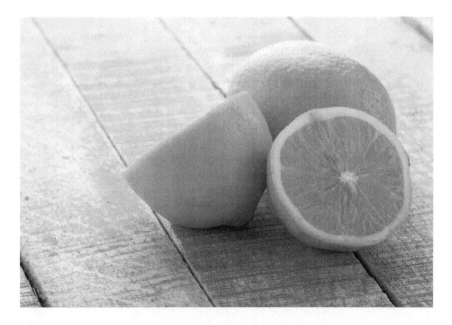

More recent research suggests that lemons may help to protect the brain and prevent strokes in women.

Eat lemons along with foods that are rich in iron to get the maximum nutritional benefit. The high Vitamin C content in the lemon will help the body to absorb and use the iron more effectively.

Add lemon juice to your drinking water, or squeeze it on fish, grains, vegetable, and chicken dishes. Always go with fresh lemons since pre-squeezed juice quickly loses its Vitamin C.

Limes

Limes contain even more Vitamin C than lemons and oranges and contain limonoid, an anti-carcinogenic compound found to be effective in preventing cancers of the breast, lung, skin, stomach, and mouth, and other types of cancers.

Vitamin C is instrumental in lowering inflammation throughout the body, and protects against heart disease, arthritis, and asthma.

Add lime juice to your drinking water as an aid in weight loss. The acidity in the juice breaks down body fat and is good for digestive problems by helping to break down carbs.

Lingonberries

Though less well known than other berries, the lingonberry offers plant polyphenols in high concentration and are an excellent natural treatment for urinary tract infections.

Lingonberries literally prevent the bacterium that causes UTIs from adhering to the walls of the bladder.

In addition to their antioxidant content, lingonberries are a good source of Vitamin A, Vitamin C, Vitamin B, calcium, and magnesium. They are excellent for lowering blood pressure and may support natural weight loss.

Mangoes

The sub-tropical mango grows primarily in Asia, Africa and South America. Rich in Vitamin C, fiber, polyphenols, and carotenoids, the mango is sometimes called the "king of all fruits."

Well regarded for strengthening the immune system, mangoes also promote weight loss and reduce signs of aging. Eat mangoes to clear up acne, heal wounds, and soothe dry, scaly skin. The beta-carotene in mangoes also reduces the damage caused by air pollutants, UV light, and environmental toxins.

Oranges

Oranges are a popular snack for their aromatic, sweet flavor and juicy consistency, but they also contain high amounts of Vitamin C, Vitamin A, antioxidants, flavonoids, potassium, calcium, magnesium, and dietary fiber.

Researchers have determined that oranges, like many citrus fruits, contain D-limonene, which provides protection against breast, lung, mouth, and skin cancer. Hesperidin in oranges combined with magnesium lowers blood pressure and reduces bad cholesterol. When hesperidin unites with pectin, it prevents the body from absorbing fat.

A glass of freshly squeezed orange juice per day helps to relieve pain from inflammatory disorders including arthritis. For men, the folate in oranges protects their sperm from genetic damage and can be an important nutritional support for couples trying to conceive a healthy baby.

Papaya

The mild papaya fruit contains a host of natural enzymes that support good digestion and work to heal a weakened or sluggish metabolism. It is an excellent weight loss aid at just 55 calories per cup and thanks to its low sugar content is appropriate for diabetics.

Papaya also has protective benefits against heart disease and cancer thanks to the presence of lycopene and beta-cryptoxanthin. Proteolytic enzymes in the fruit are anti-inflammatory, helping to soothe the pain of arthritis and osteoporosis.

(As a topical application, papaya is good for skin health and is often used in moisturizers for the face and lips.)

Peaches

Peaches are excellent snacks year round but are especially good during the hot months to provide hydration and prevent muscle cramps. They are low in calories, but high in Vitamin A, Vitamin C, beta-carotene, and lutein.

Lab studies have shown peach extract to slow the growth of breast and colon cancers, while research at the National Cancer Institute found peaches and related fruits effective in preventing cancers of the mouth, throat, or larynx.

Pineapple

Pineapples contain the enzyme bromelain, which blocks many of the metabolic processes that lead to inflammation. In isolation, bromelain has been found useful in treating sports injuries and associated swellings as well as blood clots and even digestive problems.

Pineapple is also a good source of manganese, Vitamin B1, and Vitamin C. A smoothie becomes a real dessert when pineapples are added. Pineapple are also great mixed in yogurt or added to any pork meats when roasting.

Pomegranate

From Greek mythology to ancient Egyptian burial rites, the pomegranate has been with us since ancient times. Cultivated in the Mediterranean, this delicious and unusual fruit is mentioned in the holy books of Christianity, Judaism, and Islam.

Pomegranate juice is a good source of Vitamin C, potassium, and Vitamin B5. The fruit's polyphenols and antioxidants have shown the potential to lower the risk of atherosclerosis, while its content of linoleic acid combats insulin resistance. In lab studies, pomegranate seed oil has proved to be effective against breast cancer cells.

Used topically, pomegranate seed oil stimulates keratinocytes in the outer layer of the skin to help reverse damage from the sun and aging.

It is also a powerful anti-inflammatory that absorbs deeply with no greasy residue. It can help to reduce scars, soothe minor irritations, and even improve sunburns, acne, eczema, and psoriasis.

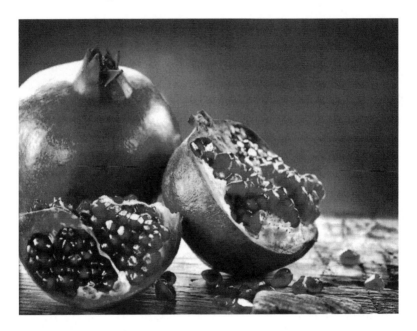

Tomatoes

Although tomatoes are filled with lutein, Vitamins A, Vitamin C, carotenes, anthocyanins, and potassium, their real "super" component is lycopene. This single substance is the best yet discovered to stop the action of free radicals and to protect the skin from aging caused by UV light.

Lycopene has the potential to combat prostate, breast, pancreatic, and intestinal cancers. It is most effective in cooked tomatoes, and when tomatoes are eaten in combination with broccoli.

Chapter 3 - The Super Veggies

The "super" vegetables listed in this chapter stand out for their high content of vitamins, fiber, and phytochemical for fighting disease. Many are members of the cruciferous (cabbage) family that are especially touted for their ability to lower the risk of developing cancer.

In 1996, the *Journal of the American Dietetic Association* published a research review regarding cruciferous vegetables. The authors found that more than 70% of the literature supported the link between these "super" foods and an anti-carcinogenic effect.

Eating a diet rich in vegetables lowers the risk of cardiovascular disease including stroke, protects against type-2 diabetes, lowers blood pressure, decreases bone loss, and supports weight loss. That's a lot of bang for very little buck in the grocery store aisle!

Artichoke

All too often the only time we encounter artichokes is in combination with spinach stirred up in a yummy but fat laden dip. Fresh artichokes, with their thick outer petals guarding the succulent inner heart are daunting and confusing for the average cook.

In truth, the artichoke is versatile and an excellent source of fiber. A medium artichoke has 10 grams, a good start on the 25 grams per day recommended for women under 50.

Artichokes also contain disease-fighting compounds called polyphenols rich in anti-inflammatory antioxidants. In 2004, the U.S. Department of Agriculture determined that artichokes are one of the best vegetables for antioxidant content, while also offering high levels of Vitamin D, Vitamin K, magnesium, potassium, and folate.

It's wasteful to just go for the heart of the artichoke and not extract the flesh from the petals. The best way to do that is to more or less rake the leaf between your teeth, scraping off the tasty flesh.

Fresh artichokes are at their prime from Mary to May. Buy those that are firm and heavy with bright green leaves. Rinse and scrub the artichoke in water, then cut off the bottom stem leaving about half an inch in place. Some cooks like to use scissors to snip the thorns off the tips of the leaves as well.

Rub the cut part of the artichoke with a lemon slice to prevent browning during cooking. Steam for 30-40 minutes. Use the petals as appetizers, and extract the heart to be used in pasta, salads, or dips.

Asparagus

Asparagus spears are an excellent source of the B vitamin, folate, which is essential for the synthesis of key mood-influencing neurotransmitters including dopamine, serotonin, and norepinephrine.

One cup of cooked asparagus contains 268 mcg of folate, a

full two-thirds of the recommended daily allowance for women. Mixed with pasta, which is fortified with folic acid (synthetic folate) and you have a real mood-enhancing, healthy meal.

Beets

The antioxidant betalains give beets their vibrant, purple pigment while warding off cancer and degenerative diseases. Beets also contain Vitamin A, Vitamin B, and Vitamin C, which manufacture red blood cells, produce collagen, and improve immune function.

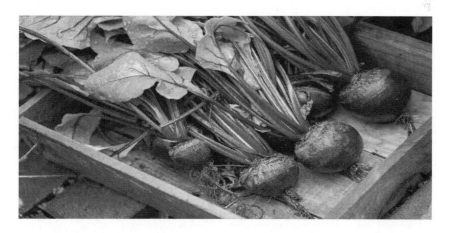

Packed with potassium, which supports digestion and vital organ function, beets are also a superb source of the B9 vitamin folate. Among its other benefits, folate reduces the risk of neural defects in babies. (It also helps to prevent graying hair!)

Since beets contain natural sugars, a single cup adds up to 58 calories with 9 grams of sugars. For this reason, diabetics should limit their intake. Prepare beets by boiling, baking, or steaming or eat them raw.

Treat the beet greens and stems as if they were spinach or Swiss chard. You can buy beets year round, but they are at their best from June to October.

Beans

Legumes are excellent for lowering cholesterol and fighting cancer while offering rich levels of fiber, folate, and magnesium. Some varieties are rich in iron with white beans having the highest concentrations.

Most beans have about 2 grams of protein per ounce, and when mixed with rice for amino acid content can easily take the place of meat in the diet. They are low in fat, cholesterol free, and calorie kind, with the "fattest" garbanzo beans adding up to no more than 33 calories per ounce.

Beans do cause flatulence because they contain an indigestible form of sugar that ferments in the large intestine and causes gas. Soak your beans to break down the sugar and drain and rinse canned beans for the same positive effect. Also, introduce beans into the diet slowly to allow the digestive system to get used to the higher levels of fiber.

Beans are both versatile and cheap, costing less than $1 a pound! (Always wash canned beans to lower the sodium content.)

Bell Peppers

Bell peppers, which originated in Mexico, are mild and sweet. They are commonly found in red, yellow, green, and orange, but can also be white, black, purple, blue, maroon, and brown. (Of all the colors, the green bell peppers are less sweet and have fewer phytochemicals.)

The peppers are a high fiber, low calorie food that also offer a sustained release of hydration since they are 93 percent water by weight. Technically a fruit, bell peppers are used as a vegetable for cooking.

Bell peppers are an excellent source of antioxidant-rich phytochemicals including chlorogenic acid (slows glucose release in the bloodstream), zeaxanthin (aids in eye health by guarding against retinal degeneration), and coumaric acid (thought to prevent prevent stomach cancer.)

They also contain high levels of Vitamin A, Vitamin C, beta-carotene, thiamine, B6, and folic acid. They bring down blood levels of homocysteine, which reduces the risk of heart attack.

Broccoli

Broccoli is a cruciferous vegetable that for many folks is a tough dietary sell. Fibrous and tough if cooked poorly, broccoli is an all-star cancer fighter, so effective, in fact, that if you're not a fan, you need to rethink your position. With high levels of Vitamin C and folate to ward of stroke and heart attack, and superb fiber content, broccoli is rich in multiple benefits. There's debate about which method of preparation best delivers that potential: raw, steamed, or boiled.

Since studies suggest that only four servings per week will ward of several cancers including prostate cancer, your best batch is to mix up the recipes and just get that broccoli in your diet, period!

Brussels Sprouts

Brussels sprouts get less attention than other superfoods, yet they contain more Vitamin C than oranges. An ounce of cooked Brussels sprouts contains 29% of the recommended daily dose, while a comparable amount of navel oranges provides only 25%. (For weight loss, an ounce of cooked Brussels sprouts contains only traces of fat and just 10 calories.)

Vitamin C is excellent for skin health and even reduces cellulite thanks to the compound indole-3-carbinol (I3C), a pre-cursor to diindolylmethane (DIM). Enzymes in DIM block the production of 16-OH estrogens that break down collagen and cause cellulite. By encouraging collagen synthesis, Vitamin C also increases vein strength.

The benefits don't stop there. Vitamin C also improves the body's ability to absorb iron, and a study at Arizona State University found that it may even help us burn fatter when we exercise.

The real hidden power of Brussel sprouts, however, lies in

their unusually high concentration of anti-carcinogenic glucosinolates -- more than any other cruciferous vegetable. When foods containing glucosinolates are chewed, they produce isothiocyanates, highly reactive mustard oils beneficial to human health.

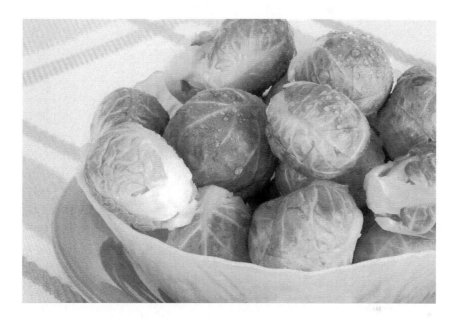

In the body the oils induce Phase II enzymes that render cancer-causing agents harmless. They also stimulate tumors to self-destruct, a process called apoptosis.

As if that single ounce of Brussels sprouts hadn't already offered enough nutritional punch, it will also give you half of the daily-recommended dose of Vitamin K your body needs. New research indicates that Vitamin K is not only fundamental for blood coagulation, but also for overall cardiovascular health.

Cabbage

We've long known that cabbage aids weight loss because it has such a high water content, but it is also an excellent source of fiber and works wonders for the stomach. Raw cabbage even helps to cure stomach ulcers.

Red cabbage contains the antioxidant anthocyanins found in blue, purple, and red plants, which reduces inflammation and improves brain function. As an added benefit, cabbage lowers cholesterol by preventing bile from absorbing fat after a meal.

Both the anthocyanins and the glucosinolates in cabbage are cancer inhibiting. Three cups or more of cabbage per week lowers the risk of breast cancer in women 50-70% according to the results of a study from Michigan State University.

Cabbage is not a "one stop shop" vegetable. It comes in several varieties, including Savoy, spring greens, green, red, and white cabbages. It's best not to overcook cabbage. Keep it crunchy! Heat breaks down some of the chemical compounds that give cabbage such a powerful health punch, including glucosinolates. Try eating cabbage raw, steamed, or lightly sautéed.

Inexpensive and readily available year round, look for tightly packed cabbage bulbs that are heavy and vivid in color. A whole cabbage refrigerated will last 1-2 weeks. Chopped cabbage goes bad in 5-6 days.

As a word of caution, too much cabbage can lead to an enlargement of the thyroid gland called a "goiter." This is rare, however, in developed countries and cooking neutralizes this potential drawback.

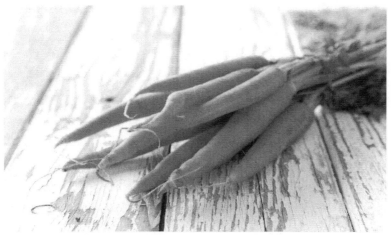

Carrots

High beta-carotene levels along with vitamins and phytochemicals give carrots their super powers. These include slowing the growth of cancer cells, especially those of the mouth, esophagus, and stomach.

Other studies indicate this list should also include cervical cancer, although more research is needed to establish this connection. Carrots do contain the natural pesticide, falcarinol, which has been found to retard tumor growth in rats.

For the highest antioxidant effect, cook your carrots, but leave them whole until they're done. This reduces nutrient loss and makes the carrots sweeter to the taste.

Edamame

Edamame are young, green soybeans that have not been dried. They are harvested in the pod and make an excellent high-fiber snack with isoflavones, and protein. All these nutrients lower the risk for cardiovascular disease while bringing down LDL cholesterol.

The isoflavones mimic estrogen, which can ease menopause symptoms. They may also increase bone density, staving off the osteoporosis with which many struggle later in life.

A half a cup of edamame offers 4 grams of fiber and 8-11 grams of protein with just 120 calories.

Hot Peppers

All peppers, regardless of how mild or hot, contain capsaicsinoids. While capsaicin gives peppers their flavor, it also fights inflammation, prevent heart disease, improves circulation, lowers blood pressure, and alleviates arthritis pain.

Peppers also contain Vitamin A, Vitamin C, and beta-carotene. All are powerful antioxidants. Considering the endless ways in which peppers can be incorporated into recipes, this is an easy superfood to work into your daily meals. Just remember, the hotter the better when it comes to health benefits!

If that fact has or is stopping you from eating foods with peppers, start with the hottest you can tolerate for now, and gradually develop your tolerance.

Kale

Many hardcore kale fanatics swear it is not "a" superfood, but "the" superfood! The point is hard to argue considering kale's resume of health benefits that include vitamins, minerals, and phytonutrients like glucosinolates and flavonoids.

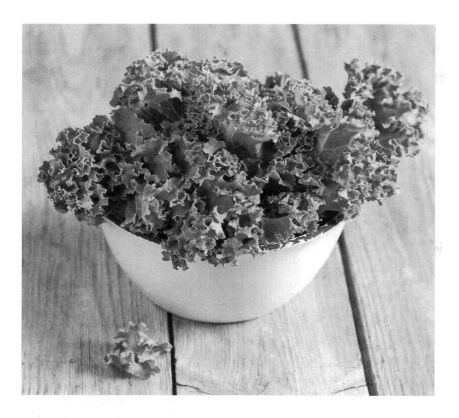

The specific glucosinolates include glucobrassicin, glucoraphanin, and sinigrin. The body converts these compounds into isothiocyanates in the digestive tract. There is strong evidence that isothiocyanates prevent cancer and may suppress tumor growth by triggering apoptosis or the self-destruction of cancerous cells.

Although the bulk of current research entails colon and breast cancer, there is good evidence to suggest these effects also apply to prostate, ovarian, and bladder cancer.

The potent combination of nutritional components in kale allows this single vegetable to combat cardiovascular disease, rheumatoid arthritis, asthma, and many cancers while promoting urinary tract health and even reversing the effects of pre-mature aging.

Kale has almost as much Vitamin A as carrots, which is known to promote healthy surface linings in the urinary tract. In a study published in 2007, Vitamin A was found to reduce the chronic UTI infection rate in a control group from 3.6 to 0.8.

At the same time, kale has low oxalate levels, and thus is a good leafy green choice for people who suffer from calcium-oxalate kidney stones.

Kale's powerhouse of antioxidants includes kaempferol and quercetin. It is one of the few vegetables to carry a high Oxygen Radical Absorbance Capacity (ORAC) rating. Others in this rarified group include raw garlic, red cabbage, sweet potatoes, Savoy cabbage, beet greens, and arugula.

The ORAC rating measures a food's ability to scavenge for free radicals, the unstable molecules that damage our bodies at the cellular level. This damage has been linked to the pathogenesis of many disease including:

- macular degeneration
- cardiovascular disorders
- thrombosis
- asthma
- immunological impairment
- atherosclerosis
- Alzheimer's disease
- diabetes
- rheumatoid arthritis

As an added benefit, the neutralization of free radicals also improves skin elasticity and repairs damage from excess exposure to ultraviolet radiation.

Eat kale raw or sauté it in a pan with chopped onions. Add a drizzle of extra virgin olive oil and you have a wonderfully satisfying and healthy warm dish.

Mustard Greens

Like many deeply hued plants, the dark purple to bright green leaves of the mustard plant contain powerful antioxidants that help to clear the body of toxins.

The sulforaphane content of mustard greens lowers cholesterol and their glucosinolates become cancer fighting and tumor suppressing isothiocyanates in the body. The effect of isothiocyanates is especially pronounced with bladder, colon, breast, lung, prostate and ovarian cancer.

Mustard greens have a peppery, slightly pungent taste and should be mixed with sweeter salad elements to make them more palatable. As an alternative, sauté the greens with onion and garlic and drizzle them with sesame oil for a tasty side dish.

Spinach

Spinach has an amazingly full resume of nutritional benefits including:

- Vitamins A, C, and K
- B Vitamins, including folate and riboflavin
- iron
- calcium
- magnesium
- manganese
- potassium
- copper
- phosphorous
- zinc
- selenium
- antioxidants
- Omega-3 fatty acids
- lutein

Cooked spinach is a better source of iron and should be served with an additional food rich in Vitamin C to enhance absorption.

People who incorporate spinach in their diets have a reduced risk of macular degeneration and cataracts and are better protected from eye damage due to sun exposure. Spinach is a high-oxalate food, however, and should be eaten in moderation by those with kidney disease, rheumatoid arthritis, and gout.

Swiss Chard

Swiss chard, which is a close relative of the beet, contains the same betacyanins, betaxanthins, and antioxidant phenols and flavonols, all of which have been shown to inhibit the growth of cancer cells. Chard also contains excellent levels of:

- Vitamins C, E, and K
- potassium
- magnesium
- iron
- manganese
- B6, thiamine, niacin, and folic acid
- calcium,
- selenium,
- zinc
- carotenes
- fiber

A single cup service has 27.4% of the recommended daily value for potassium and 47% for magnesium. (Both are instrumental in the regulation of blood pressure.)

Like many greens, Swiss chard does contain measurable oxalates. Keep your consumption low if you suffer from kidney disease, gout, or rheumatoid arthritis.

Chapter 4 – The Super Grains

There are many more grains available to us than most people realize, all of them packed with fiber, protein, vitamins, minerals, and carbohydrates. What makes these lesser-known grains really stand out, however, is that they are gluten free.

Since most experts recommend at least 6 servings of grain per day, mixing it up with flavors beyond wheat and corn and getting "super" nutritional value is a "no brainer."

Barley

Barley has twice the level of fiber and cancer-fighting selenium as the more popular brown rice and also cooks faster!

A form of barley called beta glucan helps to lower cholesterol and bring down the body's rate of fat absorption.

Brown Rice

Brown rice retains the outer bran or germ layer. As a staple in many cultures, brown rice contains excellent amounts of manganese, magnesium, selenium, and fiber.

Manganese guards against free radicals while magnesium reduces the risk for diabetes along with cardio-protective qualities. Selenium is believed to retard the development of colon cancer. Fiber lowers cholesterol and aids in weight regulation.

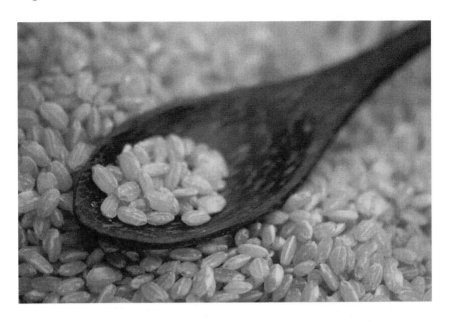

There are more than 8,000 varieties of rice in short, medium, and long grain types. It is available year round in organic form and is naturally gluten free. The largest producing countries are China, Thailand, and Vietnam.

Brown rice stored at room temperature will keep for six months; longer in the refrigerator or freezer. Cooked brown rice is good for five days if kept refrigerated.

Teff

Teff is the world's smallest grain, so tiny in fact that it can't be refined or processed. It's popular, however, due to its versatility, leading all the grains in calcium content.

White and dark teff can be purchased online or in health food stores for about $8 per pound. A single 1/4 cup serving has 160 calories.

Teff is sweeter than wheat with a flavor like molasses. Simmer one cup of teff with two cups of water covered for 20 minutes or until the liquid has been absorbed for a warm breakfast cereal. (Be sure to add fresh fruit on top.)

You can often find teff tortillas, which are great for wraps and easier to handle than the loose grain.

Millet

Millet is used around the world for bread, porridge, and beer, but in the United States it's mainly sold as birdfeed. Since millet is high in magnesium and B vitamins, that's great for the birds, but humans are missing out on an excellent source of nutrients that reduce nerve and muscle pain, alleviate migraine headaches, and help to control diabetes.

Prepare millet as a hot cereal or use millet flour for baking. Whole millet is available in health food stores for approximately $2 a pound. Choose "hulled" over "pearled." Hulled millet is whole grain and offers higher fiber content.

Kamut

Kamut contains 40% more protein than wheat, along with omega-3 fatty aides, Vitamin E, and B vitamins. This combination helps to boost the immune system while fighting inflammation in the body.

Look for kamut in ready-made pastas, baked as a bread, sold as whole grain, or ground as a flour. Regardless of form, most cost $2-$4 per pound.

Buckwheat

Buckwheat is basically allowed to come out and play with the grains even though it is not one of the family or even a wheat. Buckwheat is most closely related to rhubarb and is valuable nutritionally for its high levels of rutin, which lowers cholesterol and improves circulation.

Buckwheat is available in many forms from noodle to pancake mixes. In Japan it is called "soba," and you may also see buckwheat labeled "kasha" which means it has been toasted. Depending on the form, most products cost $3-$7.

As a replacement for rice, boil 1 cup of toasted buckwheat (kasha) with 2 cups water or broth for 10 minutes. Allow the mixture to stand for 5 minutes and then sauté with onions or vegetables for a delicious pilaf!

Oats

Oats lay claim to superfood status because they are a wholegrain complex carbohydrate high in fiber and filled with cholesterol lowering potential thanks to the presence of beta glucan.

The term "wholegrain" indicates a grain with its three layers intact: the bran, endosperm, and germ. In this form, edible grains retain the natural vitamins and minerals. Refined grains, on the other hand, are nothing but the starchy, endosperm.

The insoluble fiber in oats passes through the digestive system without being absorbed, bulking up stools for better regularity and bowel health.

The carbohydrates and fiber in oats provide good energy and make an excellent breakfast food to get the day off to a good start.

Quinoa

Quinoa exists in the nether world of the "pseudocereal." It's generally considered to be a grain, but it is more closely related to beets and spinach. Unlike wheat and other popular grains, quinoa is gluten free.

One cup of cooked quinoa has 8 grams of protein and contains all of the essential amino acids. It's also a good source of magnesium, manganese, and calcium, and contains varying amounts of Vitamin B2, Vitamin E, iron, phosphorus, copper, and zinc.

There are some potentially negative considerations with quinoa. It does have more fat than true grains and it's a source of oxalates, which can cause problems for people with a history of kidney stones.

Also, saponins in the outer covering of raw quinoa act as both a diuretic and laxative. To ameliorate these effects, rinse quinoa before cooking.

Chapter 5 – Can Animal Foods Be Super Too?

Animal foods get a bad rap in the health community, but they certainly can and do have a place in a well-balanced diet. I enjoy a primarily plant-based menu because it seems to better suit my constitution, but that does not make me blind to the nutritional benefits of animal-based foods.

According to the American Heart Association, you should limit your intake of saturated fat per day to less than 7% of your total calories consumed, and keep your daily intake of cholesterol under 300 mg. There are numerous healthy animal choices to help you manage your consumption within those limits.

Organ Meats

Organ meats are a natural multivitamin, so packed with healthy fat, essential amino acids, vitamins, and minerals that it's hard to compare them to any other food.

Once regarded as a delicacy, organ meats are not consumed in large volume in modern society, which is a huge waste of healthy potential. Even a single serving of grass-fed liver per week can significantly increase levels of iron for healthier blood and circulation.

An 8 ounce portion of grass-fed beef liver contains 250 calories compared to 306 for liver from a grain fed animal. That's even leaner than an 8 ounce portion of round steak at 361 calories. That same serving of liver has 7 grams of total fat (3 grams of saturated fat) and 545 mg of cholesterol.

Grass-fed Beef

Grass fed beef comes from cows that have grazed year round in a pasture rather than being fed a processed, grain-based diet. This makes the beef much healthier, ensuring excellent levels of omega-3 fats, Vitamin E, beta-carotene, and conjugated linoleum acid.

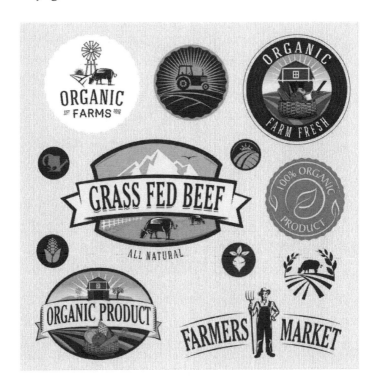

Grass-fed beef is, on average, 40-50% saturated fat, 40-50% monounsaturated fat, and 10% polyunsaturated fat.

- Saturated fats are the "bad" ones, increasing total cholesterol and increasing the risk of developing type 2 diabetes.

- Monounsaturated fats decrease the risk of breast cancer, lower cholesterol, aid in weight loss, protect us against heart disease and stroke, and reduce belly fat.

- Polyunsaturated fats are found in nuts, seeds, vegetable oils and fatty fish. These are the much touted Omega-3 and Omega-6 fatty acids which help to lower total cholesterol.

For a more precise nutritional breakdown, let's look at a 4 ounce, grass-fed, strip steak that has been cooked. This cut contains the following daily-recommended levels of the listed nutrients:

- Vitamin B12 - 60%
- Protein - 52.3%
- Vitamin B3 - 47.5%
- Omega-3 Fats - 45.8%
- Vitamin B6 - 43.5%
- Selenium - 43.5%
- Zinc - 37.1%
- Phosphorus - 34.3%
- Choline - 17.3%
- Pantothenic Acid - 15.4%

In absolute best case scenarios, the much demonized beef is 60% "good" and 40% "bad," numbers that can certainly be worked to your advantage with proper menu planning and moderation — about 2-3 servings per week.

Grass-fed beef is one of the best sources of conjugated linoleic acid, a potent antioxidant and Vitamin K2, a powerful agent against heart disease that is difficult to find in dietary sources.

Bone Broth

Bone broth is another powerful "multivitamin," especially when it's made from grass fed beef bones or healthy chicken bones. Bone broth is excellent to

- heal the gut and promote better digestion through its action as a hydrophilic colloid, attracting and holding liquid

- reduce joint pain and inflammation thanks to its high levels of glucosamine

- promote strong healthy bones as a by-product of good calcium and magnesium levels

- inhibit infections caused by the cold and flu viruses

- fight inflammation in the tissues and organs with the amino acids glycine, proline, and arginine

- promote better sleep with the amino acid glycine, which has a calming effect

- promote the growth of healthy hair and nails via its gelatin content

Bone broth can be used in any recipe or consumed as a hot drink. Incorporating even a cup a week delivers a strong nutritional punch.

Wild Salmon

In selecting fish for your diet, always choose those that are wild caught over farm-raised fish that are fed soy pellets. Salmon should be at the top of your list of high quality fish selections for its exceptional omega-3 content as well as protein, essential amino acids, calcium, iron, zinc, magnesium, phosphorus, and Vitamins A, D, B6, B, and E.

Incorporating wild salmon into your diet 1-3 times per week offers:

- protection for heart health
- reduced risk of stroke
- reduced risk of type 2 diabetes
- improved cholesterol levels
- improved blood vessel function
- improved immune function
- protection for depression and Alzheimer's

Depending on your location, you can pay as much as $15 - $20 a pound, so this healthy food may go on your list of occasional indulgences!

Eggs

Another controversial and maligned food, the rich yolk of an egg is high in the essential B vitamin choline, and contains the following recommended daily percentages of the listed nutrients:

- Vitamin A - 6%
- Folate - 5%
- Vitamin B5 - 7%
- Vitamin B12 - 9%
- Vitamin B2 - 15%
- Phosphorus - 9%
- Selenium - 22%

Eggs also have good amounts of calcium, zinc, and vitamins D, E, K, and B6.

That's all packed into a 77 calorie food (per large egg) with 6 grams of protein and only 5 grams of healthy fat.

Eggs do contain 212 mg of cholesterol, more than half of the 300 mg recommended daily intake, but the individual response to egg consumption varies widely. In 70% of people, eggs don't raise cholesterol at all, and in the other 30%, the elevation is mild.

Look for a local source for your eggs, preferably from free range chickens that get lots of sunlight.

Sardines

Although many people find the idea of eating sardines repugnant, if you can or will incorporate these tiny fish into your diet, you'll be availing yourself of a truly dense source of omega-3 fatty acids, far better than any fish oil supplement.

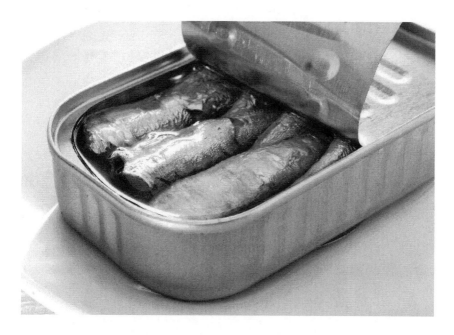

Omega-3s lower cholesterol, reduce the risk of heart disease, and help to relieve chronic inflammation — all while boosting brain function and improving your memory!

A 3.75 ounce can of sardines contains:

- 10.53 grams of fat with only 1.4 grams of unhealthy saturated fat

- 351 milligrams of calcium, 50% more than an 8 ounce glass of milk

- 2.69 milligrams of iron

- 451 milligrams of phosphorus

- 178 I.U. of Vitamin D

- And some degree of magnesium, potassium, zinc, and Vitamin B12

Sardines do carry a heavy sodium load, however, approximately 465 milligrams.

Grass-Fed Butter and Ghee

Butter as a healthy food choice? Yes, so long as it's high quality yellow butter, not white, and made from the milk of grass fed cattle. Butter is an excellent source of conjugated linoleic acid, which actually helps to reduce fat in the body while protecting against cancer and heart disease.

All grass-fed dairy items, including butter, are rich in heart-healthy Vitamin K2, and they have the optimal 1:1 ratio of omega-3 to omega-6 fatty acids.

Ghee is clarified butter with the milk solids removed. It can be used at higher temperatures for cooking and is typically better tolerated by people with a sensitivity to dairy products.

Raw Milk and Kefir

Raw milk from grass-fed cattle offers all the same benefits as those discussed above for butter. The real dietary caution in regard to dairy is avoiding "low fat" products that are actually loaded with chemicals, hormones, and sugar!

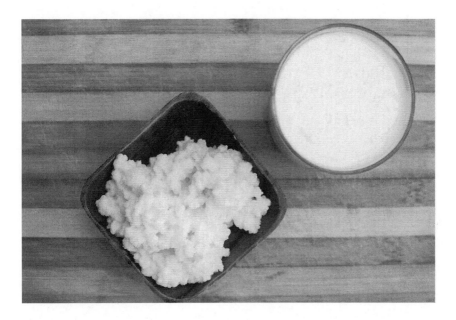

Raw milk has not been pasteurized, so basically, you'll have to have a local source and one that you trust. The purpose of pasteurization is to remove pathogenic bacteria including Campylobacter, Salmonella, and E. coli. If you can't find clean raw milk, in my opinion, you should not consume dairy.

As a bit of extra good news, if you are lactose intolerant, a recent study found that 80% of people who share your diagnosis can drink raw milk with no negative effects.

Kefir is fermented milk (cow, sheep, or goat) that contains probiotic cultures for gut health and has anti-fungal properties. Think of it as drinkable yogurt. Its reputed benefits include:

- boosting immunity
- healing inflammatory bowel disease
- building bone density
- fighting allergies
- improving lactose digestion
- killing candida yeast
- supporting detoxification

Kefir is especially rich in Vitamin B12, calcium, Vitamin K2, biotin and folate.

Chapter 6 - Additional Superfoods

The following superfoods don't fall neatly into a fruit or vegetable category, but they all offer attractive benefits including adding variety to your daily diet.

Black Soybeans

Black soybeans, not yellow and green, are the standout superfood, containing the omega-3 fatty acid, linoleic acid, which reduces the risk of heart disease and fatal blood clots (thrombosis).

Black Tea

While not as well publicized as green tea, black teas also contain phytochemicals and antioxidants to fight heart disease and guard against stroke and cancer.

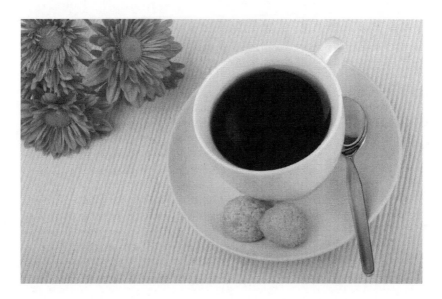

A particular phytonutrient, catechins, prevent sunburn and age spots. As an added benefit, black tea drinkers have better oral health and may have less muscle soreness from exercise.

Camu Camu

In trendy nutritional circles, the Brazilian fruit camu camu is being lauded as the "new" acai for its amazing antioxidant properties and natural energy boosting qualities.

The plant is indigenous to flooded rainforests in Peru, Brazil, Colombia, and Venezuela. In those regions camu camu leaves and fruit are used for medicinal purposes.

Among its many benefits, the light orange fruit, which is about the size of a lemon, is said to contain strong anti-viral powers in addition to high Vitamin C content. It's helpful for the common cold, cold sores, herpes and shingles.

The concentration of Vitamin C in camu camu is impressive, a single teaspoon packs in 1180% of the daily-recommended intake!

The fruit also contains a host of other beneficial substances:

- Valine, which prevents the breakdown of muscle tissue and is important to support cognitive function and the nervous system.

- Potassium, essential for proper heart and kidney

function. Every 100 grams of camu camu has 71.1 mg of potassium.

- Leucine, an essential amino acid the human body needs for the production of growth hormones, recovery, and proper muscle and bone growth.

- Serine, an amino acid that breaks down the bonds in proteins and polypeptides for proper digestion.

- Multiple flavonoids, which act as antioxidants to neutralize harmful free radicals.

- Gallic acid, which is an antioxidant, but also has anti-fungal and anti-viral properties.

- Ellagic acid, an antioxidant with anti-cancer effects. Research indicates it may also guard against diabetes.

Camu camu berries are difficult to locate, but you can purchase tablets or powder and use them to flavor other foods. Since there is some concern that the fruit can interfere with some chemotherapy medications, always talk to your doctor before taking this or any other supplement.

Chia Seed

Chia seeds come from a plant in the mint family. Approximately one ounce of the seeds contains 5 grams of protein and 10 grams of fiber. They are also an excellent source of Omega-3 fatty acids, calcium, and phosphorous.

The seeds are easily added to everything from smoothies to meatballs. Claims that chia seeds aid in weight loss and lower blood pressure have not been proven, but their other benefits makes them well worth adding to your diet.

Cacao and Cocoa

The debate over the health benefits of chocolate really has to be based on understanding the difference between "cacao" and "cocoa."

- Cacao refers to the Theobroma Cacao tree, which puts out the cacao bean.

- Cocoa is processed from the cacao bean.

The forms of cocoa and chocolate with which we are most familiar have been robbed of their antioxidants and healthy flavanols by processing.

There are, however, worse considerations. Non-organic cocoa is heavily contaminated with pesticides, fumigants, and genetically modified organisms (GMOs). Indigenous populations paid slave wages grow more than 70% of the global supply of cocoa. (Many of these workers actually are child slaves.)

The upside to spending the additional money for raw, organic cacao is that it has more than 40 times the antioxidant levels of blueberries and has the highest known plant-based supply of iron at 7.3 mg per 100 grams. That beats out beef at 2.5 mg and spinach at 3.6 mg.

The iron content is, however, non-heme and should be part of a diet rich in Vitamin C for maximum benefit. Cacao powder is excellent mixed in smoothies in combination with fruits like oranges and kiwi.

Cacao is also one of the highest plant-based sources of magnesium, a necessary mineral for good cardiovascular health and for the efficient conversion of glucose to energy for better mental focus. At the same time is elevates levels of four neurotransmitters that enhance well-being and alleviate depression: serotonin, dopamine, anandamide and phenylethylamine.

Raw cacao also has 160 mg of calcium per 100 grams, which is more than cow's milk. You can use cacao powder as the basis for a warm (or cold) chocolate drink mixed with plant-based milk, but don't use regular dairy products. They block the absorption of the cacao's rich stores of antioxidants and calcium.

Other ways to include cacao in your diet include squares of raw, organic chocolate eaten whole, or use raw organic cacao powder in your baked goods.

Coconut, Coconut Oil, Coconut Water

Coconut is an almost perfect natural food, packed with iron, magnesium, potassium, selenium, copper, zinc, and phosphorus along with fat, carbohydrates, and protein. It began to appear on the superfood "hit parade" over the last five years, first as an unlikely weight loss aid in the form of coconut oil.

Ironically, the oil contains 87% saturated fat, but as medium-chain fatty acids (MCFAs). When MCFAs enter the bloodstream, they go straight to the liver and are converted to energy. They are not stored in the body and thus boost the body's metabolism.

Nutritional experts recommend four teaspoons of the oil per day, also touting its antiviral and antibacterial effects, which are derived from lauric acid. The oil can also be applied externally for skin conditions and may be a useful dietary component for people who suffer from chronic yeast infections and thrush. Coconut combats inflammation and has been found to stimulate the growth of new brain cells.

With a growing awareness of its nutritional value, an array of coconut products are now available including coconut butter, milk, fresh pieces, dried chips, oil, and coconut water. The water, which is low in cholesterol and high in Vitamin C has more potassium than a banana. Extracted from young coconuts, the water stimulates the action of the thyroid, further supporting weight loss.

Use coconut oil for baking rather than regular butter. It's naturally sweet but contains no fructose and remains healthy when heated because it does not oxidize.

Mix coconut in cereals, or toast coconut flakes or chips as a snack food. Coconut milk and cream are excellent for people trying to stay away from dairy, but make sure you get the unsweetened version.

Coffee

Although the debate has gone back and forth on the helpful or harmful qualities of coffee, one study suggests coffee as a powerful brain tonic. Researchers tracked a group of 700 older men over a decade. Those who drank an average 3 cups of coffee a day showed significantly less mental decline than their counterparts.

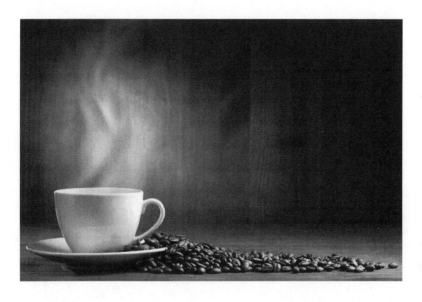

Coffee consumption has also been linked to lowered risks for Alzheimer's disease, Parkinson's, Type 2 diabetes, and colon cancer. Drinking coffee an hour before a workout can boost endurance, and the antioxidants and acids in coffee soothes inflammation. Java has been found to improve memory and to reduce heart disease by 25%.

While overdoing coffee can lead to jittery nerves and insomnia, the good news is that even decaf is good for you!

Garlic

Garlic contains the antioxidant allicin (among others) as well as manganese, selenium, Vitamins C, and Vitamin B6. The many powers attributed to garlic include both aphrodisiac and vampire repellent. There's more science to suggest, however, that garlic's real "super" qualities lie in its effects on high blood pressure, cholesterol levels, cardiovascular levels, colds, and some cancers.

- A study in 2012 determined that 200 mg of garlic powder three times a day reduces blood pressure.

- A review of 29 published studies in 2009 found that garlic powder achieves moderate reduction of cholesterol levels.

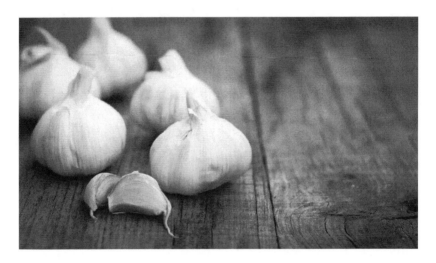

Assessments of garlic's cancer fighting abilities are mixed. In 2007 a review of available research concluded garlic possibly offers protection against stomach and bowel cancer. In 2009, however, a second review said there was no evidence to support claims for any anti-cancer properties, with the suggestion of very limited benefit against colon, prostate, oral, ovary or renal cell cancers.

Even if there are disputes about garlic's health benefits, it's important in any healthy diet as an excellent flavor alternative to salt.

Green Tea

It's hard for anyone to have missed the ongoing hype about the benefits of green tea, a staple in Asian cultures for thousands of years. The tea is believed to help control body weight while preventing cancer and heart disease.

Not all teas are the same, however. You will derive the maximum benefit from green tea by steeping the unfermented leaves in hot water. Loose green tea delivers the full effect of the phytochemical *Epigallocatechin gallate* (EGCG). It's the primary "super" component believed to fight cancer growth.

Some studies have found that green tea can block the effects of certain anti-cancer medications. If you are a cancer patient, consult with your doctor before adding the tea to your diet.

Replace your morning coffee (or at least some of it) with a cup of green tea. Two to three cups per day is recommended for maximum benefit. You'll encounter a lot of "green tea" products, but the traditional steaming cup made straight from the leaves is best.

Hemp Seeds

As a snack post-exercise or really any time, hemp seeds deliver all nine of the essential amino acids required by the body to repair tissues, build cells, and form antibodies. They're also one of the highest sources of plant-based protein available and are an excellent source of magnesium, zinc, and iron.

The entire "package" delivers protection against cancer, coronary disease, high cholesterol, and symptoms of depression. Unusually rich in gamma linoleic acid, a polyunsaturated fatty acid, hemp seeds can help allergies and improve attention deficit disorder.

An ounce of hemp seed (roughly the equivalent of two tablespoons) contains 10 grams of protein and 77% of the daily-recommended level of Vitamin E.

Lentils

Lentils are inexpensive legumes that are a cheap source of high protein (more than beef). Even hardcore carnivores will be surprised, however, by the lentil's versatility and its health benefits.

Fewer than 10% of Americans eat lentils and don't realize their powerful ability to decrease inflammation while delivering many essential nutrients including folate, iron, and potassium.

The high iron content staves off anemia in vegetarians and

vegans, while the low glycemic content of lentils prevents the kind of sudden blood sugar spikes seen with other starches.

Lentils, and in fact all grains and legumes, are good for weight loss. Eating legumes staves off hunger for an extra 2-4 hours and lentils are rich in soluble dietary fiber (three times more than bran flakes) for cholesterol reduction.

To prepare lentils rinse them under cold water and then boil for 30 minutes or less. Make sure the lentils are fully cooked to avoid gastric distress.

Lucuma

Lucuma, (pronounced loo-koo-mah) is a natural sweetener sometimes called "nature's caramel." The Peruvian fruit is so popular in its native region it is the number one ice cream flavor, beating out vanilla and chocolate.

Most readily available as a powder, lucuma lends a caramel note to anything with which it is mixed, including smoothies, baked goods, and ice creams. (Note that cooking does lower lucuma's nutrient density.)

When used as a natural sweetener, lucuma is low on the glycemic scale and imparts a subtle, sweet flavor. It's full of antioxidants including beta carotene as well as fiber, niacin, zinc, calcium and iron.

Maca Powder

Maca is a root herb that grows at altitudes of more than 12,000 feet in the Andes Mountains. It is the world's highest altitude food herb, exposed to intense sun and extreme cold.

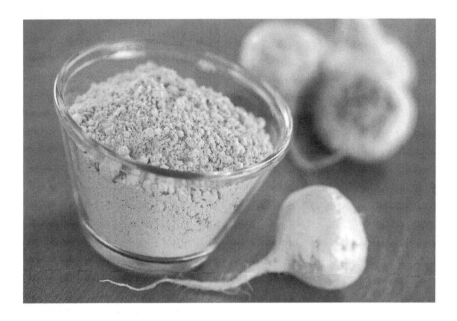

A legendary supper food of Incan warriors, maca is rich in Vitamins B1, B2, C and E and is packed with minerals:

- calcium
- magnesium
- phosphorous
- potassium
- sulfur
- iron

The herb contains traces of:

- zinc
- iodine
- copper
- selenium
- bismuth
- manganese
- silica

Maca contains almost 20 amino acids, seven that are essential, along with nearly 60 phytochemicals. When dried, maca is 60% carbohydrates, 9% fiber, and approximately 10% protein.

Most importantly, however, maca is an adaptogen, tailoring its effects to your metabolism. It has the ability to stabilize all of the body's systems, providing energy where it is needed without overstimulation.

Adaptogens increase overall vitality by 10-15%, improving the body's adaptability to stress and challenges while boosting immunity.

For nutritional use, maca powder is typically blended into drinks and smoothies. The taste is described as "earthy" with nutty overtones.

Maqui

The maqui wineberry, grown in far South America is sometimes called the "Patagonia Super Fruit," hailed primarily for its high antioxidant levels. The Mapuche Indians have eaten the small purple fruit for generations as a fermented beverage.

Maqui contains 300% more anthocyanins and 150% more polyphenols any other food or drink, including wine, making it a remarkable anti-inflammatory, anti-viral, anti-bacterial, and anti-cancer superfood.

Growing and thriving in harsh climates gives the maqui its store of UV-protectant phytochemicals, which forestall damage to the skin from toxins, pollution, and sun exposure.

Maqui has bumped acai berries from the superfood throne, earning a rating of 820 on the antioxidant scale to acai's 160-300. (The humble blackberry scores a measly 61.)

The maqui berry tastes very much like the blackberry, however, and can be added to the diet in a number of ways. Regardless of how you ingest maqui, the list of benefits are impressive and highly desirable:

- 3-4 times more antioxidants than acai or goji berries
- prevents a buildup of cholesterol
- increases insulin production
- enhances focus and energy
- curbs cravings for food by stabilizing blood sugar

For general well-being, weight loss, and anti-aging, the maqui berry is hard to beat.

Mesquite

Like many plants that grow in the desert, the mesquite's nutrients are concentrated in the tree's seeds. When ground into a powder, mesquite has high levels of magnesium, potassium, iron, calcium, zinc, fiber, and proteins. Mesquite powder can be used in flour (its gluten free) or as a seasoning. It tastes like a blend of cinnamon, chocolate, and coffee and, although sweet to the taste, is low on the glycemic index

For use as flour, combine 10-20% mesquite by weight with coconut flour or almond flour for the most flavorful and healthy results. As a spice, you can sprinkle mesquite on virtually anything, but it pairs especially well with cacao in smoothies.

Mushrooms

Mushrooms, though sometimes relegated to a low nutritional position, are excellent for lowering the risk of both heart disease and cancer. Mushrooms have no fat, sugar, or salt, but are rich in fiber, thiamine, riboflavin, niacin, pyridoxine, folate, potassium, copper, phosphorous, iron, and selenium (a rarity in fruits and vegetables.)

Since they are 90% water, adding mushroom to a dish helps it to be more filling without boosting total calorie count. There's certainly enough variety in the world of the mushroom to accommodate any cuisine, with more than 2,500 varieties.

Different mushrooms may offer different nutritional benefits. For instance, the shitake mushroom contains lentinan, an active antiviral compound that boosts the immune system. Shitake mushrooms may also help to lower cholesterol and diminish the negative effects of saturated fat.

Maitake mushrooms are an exceptional source of beta-glucans that have anti-tumor properties, while tree ear mushrooms thin the blood and help to prevent stroke and heart disease.

White mushrooms have 12-times more L-Ergothioneine than wheatgerm. A powerful antioxidant, L-Ergothioneine protect's the body's DNA from damage by free radicals. White mushrooms may also lower the risk of breast cancer.

Onions

Onions, like leeks, garlic and shallots, are part of the allium family. Packed with antioxidants, they are antiviral, antibiotic, and anti-inflammatory (thanks to high levels of quercetin).

Quercetin also offers anti-allergic qualities and may be useful in relieving asthma and hay fever by soothing inflammatory responses in the airways.

An impressive number of published studies have demonstrated the protective effects of onions against stomach cancer, a benefit that may also carry over to prostate and esophageal cancer.

In Vidalia, Georgia, home of the Vidalia onion, the death rate from stomach cancer is 50% lower than the national mortality level. The theory is that onions contain diallyl sulfide, which causes the body to produce more of the cancer-fighting enzyme glutathione-S-transferase.

Onions also help build strong bones by increasing calcium levels in the body and inhibiting the action of bone-destroying osteoclasts. The popular osteoporosis drug Fosamax works much the same way, but the onions have no side effects beyond possible bad breath.

Onions contain a range of healthy compounds including thiosulfinates, sulfides, and sulfoxides. These sulfides bring down blood lipids and regulate blood pressure. Their ability to reduce death from coronary heart disease by 20% is on par with other superfoods including broccoli, tea and apples.

Pistachios

Pistachios deserve their place on any list of superfoods as a healthy snack that is cholesterol free and high in both fiber and protein. A single ounce of these crunchy, earthy nuts gives you as much potassium as a small banana. Ongoing research suggests that pistachios bring down levels of LDL cholesterol and have excellent levels of antioxidants.

You're better off to work for this treat. People who buy pre-shelled pistachios take in 41% more calories! Eat the nuts straight out of the shell, or use them as a salad topper or an added ingredient to basil pesto. Limit yourself to about 45 nuts per serving, roughly one ounce.

Potatoes

Long shunned by dieters as "fattening" the inexpensive and versatile potato may well be "the" superfood. Offering 5.5 times more fiber than a banana and containing as much Vitamin C as three avocados, eating potatoes twice a day lowers blood pressure and contributes to weight *loss*, not gain.

Packed with vitamins, minerals, and nutrients, the potato is the central player in Dr. John McDougall's book, *The Starch Solution: Eat the Foods You Love, Regain Your Health, and Lose the Weight for Good!*, which advocates a plant-based, starch-centric diet for maximum health benefits.

Pumpkin

A pumpkin's bright orange skin signals the gourd is packed with beta-carotene, which converts to Vitamin A in the body to boost immunity, improve eye health, and prevent cardiovascular disease. Researchers also believe that the high levels of phytosterols in the seeds can reduce cholesterol and prevent cancer. These benefits can even be derived from canned pumpkin. A single cup contains 3 grams of protein and 7 grams of fiber with only 1 gram of fat and 80 calories total.

Pumpkin seeds are a treasure house of protein, magnesium, potassium, and zinc. They block prostate gland enlargement, lower the risk for bladder stones, and are a natural anti-depressant.

Pumpkin in all forms is easily added to your diet. If you do use fresh pumpkin, save the seeds and toast them in a 160-170 F oven for 15-20 minutes to create a satisfying, crunchy snack.

Red Wine

Although the red wine debate has gone back and forth for years, the most recent research indicates that 30 grams of alcohol per day, the equivalent of a large glass of red wine, cuts the risk of heart attack by half. Increasing consumption beyond that level raises the risk of cancer, and the benefit is not equal for all types of alcohol.

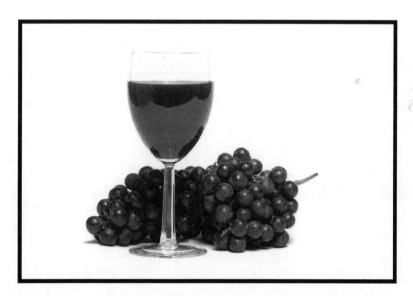

Red wine is a good choice because it also decreases LDL cholesterol, increases HDL cholesterol, thins the blood, decreases clotting, and improves digestion.

All of these positives are tied to the phytonutrients in red wine including flavonoids and resveratrol, both antioxidants. Resveratrol also inhibits the growth of cancer cells and is useful for fighting diabetes, obesity, and aging.

The recommended intake for men is two five-ounce glasses per day and one for women. If you drink more than that, you lose the antioxidant effects. But even though that may not be enough wine to qualify you as the life of the party, there's an additional upside.

A study at Columbia University found that moderate drinkers have better mental acuity than people who don't drink at all!

Seaweed

Seaweed is most familiar to Westerners in sushi rolls, but this member of the algae family, which comes in brown, red, and green varieties is an excellent source of vitamins, antioxidants, and calcium.

The most commonly eaten types are brown, mainly kelp and wakame, followed by nori, which is red.

Seaweed is used in many Asian countries, but has been elevated to a culinary art form by the Japanese, who rely on more than 20 different species. Generally, however, the serving sizes of seaweed are not large enough to deliver really impressive nutritional results.

The real reason to incorporate seaweed in your diet is its

high content of iodine, a nutrient missing in almost all other foods. Iodine is critical for good thyroid health. If this single gland in the neck is not working to produce and regulate hormones as it should, the body experiences muscle weakness and fatigue as well as rising cholesterol levels.

Since the 1920s, iodine has been added to salt in the United States. In 1993, the World Health Organization adopted a global salt iodization program.

Unfortunately, iodine-deficiency is once again becoming a common dietary problem due to three primary factors:

- health consciousness that advocates lowered salt use
- iodine-blocking chemicals in the environment
- poor quality salt used in processed foods

One gram of brown seaweed has 5-50 times the recommended-daily intake of iodine. At the same time that it is delivering this impressive benefit, seaweed also regulates levels of estrogen and estradiol to lower the risk of breast cancer, control the symptoms of PMS, and improve female fertility.

The high antioxidant content of seaweed prevents the inflammation that opens the door for a myriad of conditions including arthritis and celiac.

It's important to use seaweed in moderation. Two tablespoons of the red seaweed dulse has 34 times the amount of potassium as a banana. That's enough to cause heart palpitations in people with kidney problems. Strive for one service of brown seaweed per week that equals two tablespoons.

(Don't worry if you have several sushi rolls per week. Nori has lower iodine content than other seaweed varieties.)

Remember that seaweed originating from contaminated waters will be filled with the same toxic elements. The U.S. Food and Drug Administration strictly regulate commercial seaweed sales, but the agency does not regulate supplements. If you take seaweed pills and you don't know where the seaweed was harvested, you are taking a risk.

Shiitake Mushrooms

The shiitake mushroom is considered a gourmet delicacy, but it is also one of the most medicinal of all available mushroom varieties. Shiitakes have a rich flavor that is delicious when steamed or marinated, which are the best way to prepare these healthy "shrooms."

The heat releases not only the flavor, but also the polysaccharide rich nutrients in the shiitake. The mushrooms have a strong antiviral effect due to the presence of interferons, which inhibit the growth of pathogens like including viruses, bacteria, parasites, and even cancer.

An active component in shiitake mushrooms called lentinan stimulates and strengthens the immune response, lower cholesterol, and regulate blood pressure. Some research indicates that simply eating one mushroom a day for a week will bring serum cholesterol down 12%. Over time, that benefit rises to 40%.

The polysaccharides in shiitake mushrooms are a long-burning source of fuel for the body that protects and lubricates nerves while inhibiting tumor cells.
As if these positive weren't sufficient to send you to the store for shiitakes, they also contain iron, a host of B vitamins, Vitamin A, Vitamin D, Vitamin D, and all eight essential amino acids – a better ratio than meat and dairy foods.

Sunflower Sprouts

Sunflower sprouts qualify as a superfood not only for their nutritional value but because they can be produced in high volume and enjoyed as a salad ingredient. They have dense, thick leaves that are tasty and nourishing with high concentrations of:

- vitamins and minerals
- protein-rich amino acids
- fatty acids
- sugars
- chlorophyll

As the seeds sprout, they become nutritionally activated. The starches break down into simpler carbohydrates. Fats become fatty acids. Proteins become amino acids. All the nutrients are thus more bio-available to us when eaten.

Use sunflower seeds in the shell from the "black oil

sunflower" plant for your sprouts. Place them in a large open-mouthed jar about half full of water. The seeds will float to the top.

Seal the jar and allow the seeds to soak for eight hours. When they have doubled in size and the sprout has begun to emerge, rinse the seeds again and return to the jar in fresh water.

Cover the jar and let it sit for 1-3 days in a cool room with no direct sunlight. Rinse them again and return them to the jar for an additional 1-2 days. When the leaves have formed a "V" shape, the sprouts are ready to eat.

Sweet Potatoes

With their tasty orange flesh, sweet potatoes are one of the

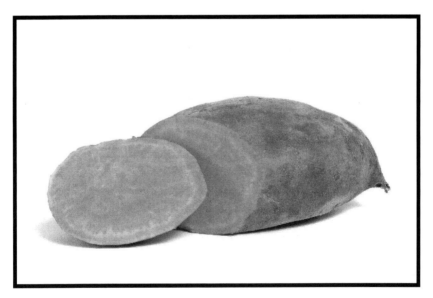

best food sources of beta-carotene. Three to 3.5 ounces per

day have the capacity to meet the daily-recommended intake of Vitamin A from 35-90%.

Sweet potatoes with purple flesh are packed with the anthocyanins, peonidins and cyanidins. Both are important as antioxidants and anti-inflammatories and are especially effective against heavy metals and oxygen radicals in the digestive tract.

To preserve the effect of the anthocyanins in cooking, be sure to steam your sweet potatoes. Boiling returns a lower glycemic index value for better blood sugar effects.

Walnuts

Walnuts are loaded with Omega 3 fatty acids and are a rich source of Vitamin B, Vitamin E, calcium, manganese, potassium, and protein. As a component of your diet, they will improve brain function, curb food cravings, and aid weight loss.

A handful of walnuts per day lowers LDL cholesterol and acts as a natural anti-depressant and anti-anxiety agent. Walnuts also regulate blood sugar and possess both antioxidant and anti-inflammatory properties.

Water

Water makes up two-thirds of the human body. Our brains are 95% water, which accounts for 82% of the blood in our veins. If the body's water supply drops by just 2% our . . .

- short-term memory gets fuzzy

- basic math skills deteriorate
- ability to focus on short print diminishes

Most daytime fatigue can be explained by mild dehydration, which plagues 75% of Americans at any one time.

The body cannot work without water, which serves as a lubricant in digestion and gives the action of joints and cartilage greater fluidity. The water in saliva facilitates chewing and swallowing, while the seat glands control over-heating through the original evaporative cooling – perspiration.

Stay well hydrated creates the foundation for all foods, super or not to function, so when in doubt? Drink another glass of water!

White Tea

New research indicates white tea reduces your risk for developing cancer and rheumatoid arthritis and takes care of pesky age-related wrinkles in the process.

In addition to high antioxidant levels, white tea stops enzymes from breaking down elastin and collagen in the skin. More significantly, however, these same enzymes, in concert with oxidants, are linked to inflammatory diseases.

Yacon

Yacon root is a prebiotic that serves as food for probiotics and good bacteria in the body. This tuber grows in the foothills of the Andes Mountains in the Amazon and has a sweet flavor similar to a smoky apple.

Due to high levels of inulin and fructooligosaccharides, yacon makes an excellent low-calorie natural sweetener safe for use by diabetics.
Yacon has diuretic properties that help flush toxins out of the body through the kidneys and in the process, lowers the risk of developing kidney stones.

Dried yacon root is an energy and brain-boosting mid-day snack. Although it can be eaten raw, yacon may cause gas in sensitive digestive systems, so consider incorporating the root in baked goods with dried fruits and nuts.

Powdered yacon root can be easily added to your morning cereal or mixed in with juice, while yacon syrup is very like dark molasses and can be used in similar ways.

Buy small amounts of either the powder or syrup. The powder must be kept dry or it tends to get sticky, and the syrup spoils easily once exposed to oxygen.

Chapter 7 - Super Herbs

Whether thought of as "medicine" or as additional nourishment, herbs offer a way to incorporate nutrients into the diet to offset dietary deficiencies. These may arise from matters of taste, lack of availability, or poor environmental quality.

For centuries, herbs have served as a vital part of folk culture, and they are an excellent adjunct to a healthy diet either as cooking ingredients or as supplements. Some super herbal "standouts" include the following.

Nettle

Nettle or "stinging nettle" has long been regarded as one of nature's best laxatives. The leaves can be dried and eaten, and are believed to aid in weight loss. One of the most popular ways of consuming nettle, however, is in tea.

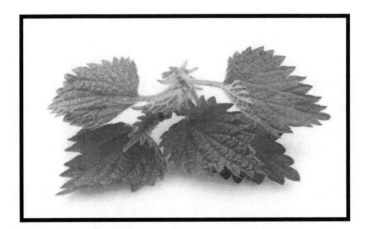

The list of purported benefits for nettle tea is long and impressive and includes the following benefits:

- stimulate the lymph system for improved immunity
- relieve arthritis symptoms
- support adrenal and thyroid function
- relieve menopause symptoms
- lower blood pressure
- reduce inflammation
- soothe nausea
- improve digestion

Check with your doctor before drinking nettle tea since there have been some reported interactions with pharmaceuticals (especially diabetes medications). Pregnant or breast feeding mothers, and people with kidney disorders should avoid nettle.

Aloe Vera

The perennial succulent aloe vera grows wild in tropical and sub-tropical climates. Research has identified seventy-five healing compounds in the plant including natural steroids, antibiotic agents, amino acids, minerals, and enzymes.

Aloe vera is most often used as a topical ointment for burns, cuts, rashes, and blemishes. Its curative powers are traced to high levels of natural sulphur (MSM), and it is also an excellent skin moisturizer.

Aloe vera juice can be used as a curative drink as well, but is best mixed with some other kind of juice to thin the consistency. Used in this way, it reduces stomach acid to improve indigestion, acid reflux, heartburn and ulcers. Other reputed benefit of the juice include:

- relief of constipation
- regulation of blood sugars
- detoxification of the body and colon
- increased metabolism for better calorie burn
- improved circulation
- lowered blood pressure
- retardation of cancer growth
- reduced inflammation
- strengthened immunity

Drink no more than 2-4 ounces per day to avoid overly loose stools.

Echinacea

Traditionally, Echinacea is used to prevent colds and flu. The herb stimulates the immune system and works as a natural antibiotic. Taking it before cold and flu season will help you to build up your resistance to infection by stimulating the flow of lymph in the body, which parallels the bloodstream and removes toxins. Echinacea is also beneficial for:

- urinary tract infections
- yeast infections
- gum disease

- tonsillitis
- strep infections
- chronic fatigue syndrome
- acid indigestion
- migraines
- various cancers (made as a tea)

Echinacea is available in capsule and liquid forms. To ward of colds and flu, begin using Echinacea 2-3 weeks in advance of the "season."

Ginseng

Ginseng helps to manage stress and relieves fatigue. It is used in Asia as an energizing tonic and is especially useful during periods of recovery from illness or surgery.

Researchers believe this effect is related to ginseng's ability to improve the body's utilization of oxygen while stimulating the metabolism. Additionally, ginseng tea improves concentration and mental abilities.

Studies have also shown that ginseng regulates blood sugar levels and is a powerful aid in managing type 2 diabetes. The extract of ginseng berries works as a natural appetite suppressant for better with weight loss.

Ginseng also eases the pain of menstrual cramps and is used as a remedy for erectile dysfunction in Asia.

Capsaicin

Although capsaicin is available as a capsule and even as a cream when used to treat arthritis pain, the compound is readily available in all forms of hot chilies. As discussed earlier in the book, it's incredibly easy to work more of these tasty fruits into your meals.

As part of your diet, the capsaicin in peppers increases body temperature. This shifts oxidation away from carbohydrates to fat for better weight loss. Capsaicin also makes you feel full faster, so you eat less.

Capsaicin lowers the risk of skin, colon, and prostate cancers, and appears to suppress the appetite since people who eat chilies regularly consume fewer calories.

The chemical structure of capsaicin excites pain-sensitive nerve endings, which is why peppers feel as if they burn when you eat them or get the juice on your skin. The affected neurons release the neurotransmitter Substance P, which transmits the sensation of pain to the brain.

As a natural pain reliever, capsaicin depletes Substance P, thus lowering the number of pain signals sent to the brain. As a cream, capsaicin can alleviate much of the discomfort of arthritis, sore muscles, and nerve pain.

Nutmeg

Nutmeg isn't just the brown powder sprinkled on top of your holiday egg nog. It's a powerful antibacterial as well as a rich, aromatic spice and is associated with a number of potential health benefits.

- better sleep
- a stronger immune system
- improved skin (as a scrub with water or honey)
- improved appearance of scars if applied topically
- a natural acne remedy
- improved digestion
- toothache relief (when used as an oil)
- enhanced mental function
- reduction of muscle and joint pain (topical application)
- strengthening of the liver

Nutmeg contains key minerals including potassium, calcium, iron, and manganese. Dust this healthy spice on various foods, including a glass of warm milk before bedtime.

Cumin

Cumin has an earthy, warm taste that lends wonderful flavor to Indian curries, Middle Eastern dishes, and chili powder. The spice can be purchased ground or in seed form. It is often used as a spice in tacos or as a meat rub.

Cumin has potent antioxidant and anti-inflammatory properties that help stop the growth of tumors. It is also believed to:

- aid digestion
- strengthen the immune system
- improve respiratory disorders
- help the common cold
- clear up skin problems
- guard against diabetes
- enhance lactation in nursing mothers
- combat anemia
- prevent or resolve hemorrhoids
- increase circulation
- improve cognitive function
- speed up the metabolism

Like many of the healthy herbs in this section, cumin is a wonderful spice to support overall health and well-being due to its broad range of potential benefits.

Turmeric

The bright yellow spice turmeric, related to ginger, is found in many Indian dishes and is responsible for the familiar color of mustard. Turmeric is made from the root of the curcuma longa plant and derives its powerful potential as a superfood from the antioxidant curcumin.

In traditional Indian medicine, turmeric is used as an anti-inflammatory to relieve pain and swelling, fight infection, and cure digestive problems. Turmeric is believed to help irritable bowel syndrome, autoimmune disorders, arthritis and tendonitis and to prevent heart disease and cancer.

When these traditional applications were put to the test in the laboratory, turmeric showed the potential to not only slow the growth of cancer cells, but to make chemotherapy more effective by protecting healthy cells from radiation damage.

Typically available as a powdered spice, turmeric oil is an effective antifungal when applied topically. A pinch of the powder applied to minor cuts works as a disinfectant and will stop bleeding. Mixed into a paste with plain water, turmeric helps to clear up acne.

Turmeric lends its bright yellow color to food while imparting an earthy tang. It's popular in curries and dishes with beans and rice. For even higher antioxidant benefits, pair turmeric with black pepper.

Heat does not reduce turmeric's beneficial effects and actually makes the curcumin more bioavailable.

Cinnamon

Cinnamon is both aromatic and tasty. Nothing smells more warm and inviting on a cold day than something baking in the oven heavily laced with cinnamon. But at the same time that your mouth is watering at the thought of those fresh cinnamon rolls, you're also about to eat a super spice with impressive health benefits.

- One-half teaspoon of cinnamon per day will lower cholesterol.

- The same amount brings down blood sugar levels and increases insulin production to assist with managing type 2 diabetes.

- Research has found that cinnamon reduces the proliferation of leukemia and lymphoma cancer cells.

- The spice has an anti-clotting effect on the blood.

- It is both an anti-fungal and an anti-bacterial. Food laced with cinnamon will keep longer, making the spice a natural preservative.

Just smelling cinnamon improves memory and cognitive function, and the spice is a natural headache and migraine remedy.

Ginger

The root ginger is a zesty spice with a long reputation in alternative medicine as an anti-inflammatory praised for supporting stomach health. Ginger has been used to treat a wide range of ailments including:

- nausea
- diarrhea
- upper respiratory infections
- hair loss
- burns

One half to one gram of ginger soothes nausea from chemotherapy, and can be useful against motion sickness.

Eating raw ginger or taking it in capsule form relieves muscles soreness and lessens the painful symptoms of arthritis. The high antioxidant content of the root may also slow the growth of cancer cells.

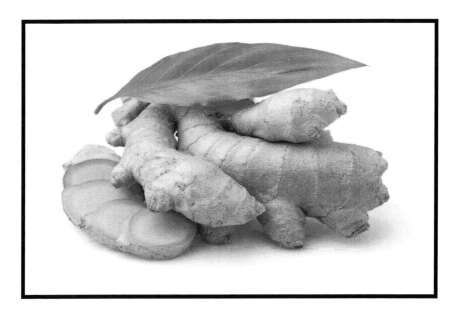

Form does alter ginger's beneficial properties. The dried powder works best for cooking, although the flavor can be overwhelming if used in excess. Use a dash of lemon or honey to soften the pungent taste.

Beware of some forms of ginger. The candied variety has been cooked in syrup and is full of sugar, while pickled ginger, often seen at the sushi counter, can have as much as 160 mg of sodium per 0.5 grams.

Sage

The herb sage is a member of the mint family and comes from an evergreen shrub. It has a sweet, savory flavor that compliments many meat dishes. In addition to its pleasant and versatile taste, sage lowers cholesterol and blood pressure and reduces the risk of heart disease.

A rich source of antioxidants, sage helps to improve memory function even with patients suffering from the opening stages of Alzheimer's. It also:

- alleviates stomach pains
- improves menstrual pain
- treats asthma
- helps in diabetes management
- reduces excessive sweating

In people who are suffering from a diminished appetite due to illness or medical treatment, the taste of sage will often encourage them to begin to eat.

Peppermint

Peppermint is an excellent source of Vitamin C and A, and is an all-purpose dietary supplement (as an oil or capsule) used to:

- ease the discomfort of indigestion
- improve irritable bowel syndrome
- combat nausea
- stop vomiting and morning sickness

- alleviate cramping in the gastrointestinal tract
- stop diarrhea
- relieve gas

As a skin preparation, peppermint oil can help to relieve headaches, muscle pains, toothaches, and rashes. It's even a natural mosquito repellent. The vapor from the oil eases congestion and coughs associated with colds and upper respiratory conditions.

Find candy made from genuine peppermint oil with no artificial flavorings and enjoy it as a healthy sweet treat!

Chapter 8 - Does How I Cook My Food Matter?

Raw food adherents would have you believe that any cooking method has a debilitating effect on the nutritional effectiveness of food. This simply isn't true. Some vegetables, like tomatoes, have higher antioxidant levels (in this case lycopene) when they are cooked. Other foods, like artichokes, can be prepared any way you like without altering their antioxidant benefits in the slightest.

Microwave

Although many people are against microwave ovens, one study conducted in Spain found that cooking vegetables in the microwave was the best way to retain nutrient content. The one exception is cauliflower, which loses 50% of its antioxidants when "nuked."

Griddle

Use your griddle for beets, celery, onions, Swiss chard, and green beans. For this group of vegetables the griddle completely preserves antioxidant content and nutritional value. Be cautious about griddles coated with non-stick chemicals that will, over time, flake off and contaminate your food. Shop for an uncoated griddle or use a thick frying pan well heated with no oil.

Grilling

The grill is a great method to get maximum nutritional value with no flavor sacrifice. You do not need much if any added fats, and if you like a smoky flavor to meats and vegetables, the grill is the place for you. Research does point to an increased risk of pancreatic and breast cancer with routine consumption of charred, well done meat, so stick with lean cuts and less cooking time.

Baking

You can bake artichokes, asparagus, broccoli, and peppers to preserve nutritional value, but surprisingly baking should *not* be used for carrots, Brussels sprouts, leeks, cauliflower, peas, zucchini, onions, beans, celery, beets, or garlic. All lose beneficial effects after time in the oven. On the flip side, however, green beans, eggplant, corn, Swiss chard, and spinach gain in nutritional value when baked.

Frying

It's somewhat ironic that the word "frying" begins with an "F," because that's the grade this cooking method earns. Frying adds too much fat to any meal and causes all vegetables to lose 5-50% of their nutritional potential. Simply put, frying is out.

Pressure Cooking and Boiling

Water is not your friend when it comes to preserving the nutritional profile of vegetables. Almost all are susceptible to partial or complete loss of antioxidant, vitamin, and mineral loss when boiled. If you have to boil your vegetables, save the water and use it in a sauce or soup to gain back that valuable content.

The only vegetable that can actually benefit from boiling is the venerable carrot. A study conducted in Ireland in 2008 found that boiling carrots increased their content of carotenoid, which boosts the immune system and contributes to healthy cardiovascular function.

Steaming

Steaming is a real winner when it comes to preparing broccoli and zucchini. For other vegetables, if you opt to steam, toss in a small amount of olive oil to boost nutrient absorption. Many vegetables contain vitamins and nutrients that are fat soluble and will be better absorbed in the presence of moderate amounts of healthy fat.

Poaching

Poaching is a close cousin of boiling. Essentially you are giving the food a small amount of time in hot water that is below its boiling point. This can increase nutrient retention, and works well for delicate foods like fish, eggs, and fruit, but don't wander too far beyond these items for this method of preparation. Poaching is really just "boiling lite."

Sautéing

Sautéing vegetables compares favorably with microwaving. This methods allows the veggies to cook in high heat for a short amount of time, which minimizes the loss of nutrients. Some people sauté food in oil, opting for healthy fat content, but water sautéing is just as effective in a cooking sense and adds no unwanted fat to your meal.

Make this decision in relation to whatever you might be pairing with your veggies to manage fat within healthy levels.

Don't Cook at All!

We really do have to give the raw food folks a nod — mostly an approving one. Raw diets have gained tons of positive press, and there are certainly compelling reasons to incorporate some raw content in a healthy diet. For one thing, if you are someone who craves a crunchy texture, it's much better to bite into a crisp vegetable than to dive into a bag of chips.

Eating raw ensures that you are not getting added fats or sugars, while capitalizing on fiber intake. It is important to remember, however, that the nutrients in some food become more bioavailable with cooking.

If you are interested in eating raw, there's more than enough literature on the subject. Get educated before you go all raw to ensure that the foods you select are giving you the right combination of nutrients delivered to their fullest potential.

Chapter 9 - Ideas for Using Your Superfoods

Throughout the text of this book, I've discussed various ways to use or incorporate your superfoods into your diet. Rather than risk those passages staying buried in the text, I've pulled out a few to highlight here.

Apricots / Granola

Fruit is one of the easiest superfoods to work into your diet because you can always put it on top of your breakfast cereal or just enjoy the fruit itself as a snack. Pairing fruit with homemade granola also gives you the opportunity to use some of the "super" grains I've discussed.

Granola is really little more than toasted oats to which you add nuts, fruits, spices, and perhaps some honey. Basic recipes, which are easily found online, call for about 3 cups of rolled oats, to which you can add other grains like kamut or barley in half-cup portions. Throw in half a cup of apricots for good measure and don't forget the ground cinnamon!

Find any basic recipe and adapt it for you new knowledge of superfoods. After 30 minutes of baking on a cookie sheet in a 300 F oven, you'll have a healthy, homemade "super" breakfast cereal.

(Don't neglect the potential to use fresh blackberries or cranberries with your granola and cereals. Both are also excellent in relishes and sauces.)

A Different Breakfast Cereal

If you'd like to try a different hot breakfast cereal, why not cook up some teff? It's much sweeter than wheat, with a flavor not unlike molasses.

Simmer one cup of teff with two cups of water covered for 20 minutes or until the liquid has been absorbed for a warm breakfast cereal.

Simple Artichokes

Don't be intimidated by the thorny looking artichoke. They're much easier to handle than you might think! Rinse and scrub the artichoke in water.

Cut off the bottom stem leaving about half an inch in place. As an option, you can use kitchen shears to also snip off the tips or "thorns" on the individual petals.

Using a lemon slice to rub the cut part of the artichoke to prevent browning during cooking. Steam for 30-40 minutes. Use the petals as appetizers, and extract the heart to be eaten as it or in pasta, salads, or dips

Easy Baked Asparagus

Like artichokes, you should not be intimidated by spears of asparagus. The best way to cook this healthy vegetable and preserve all its nutrient content is simple baking. Preheat your oven to 400 F. Arrange your asparagus on a baking sheet lightly coated so your veggies won't stick. Season to taste. Twelve minutes later, you'll have tender, delicious — and healthy — asparagus ready to serve solo or with pasta.

(Beets are another excellent baked vegetable, and you can use the greens and stems in your salad as if they were spinach or Swiss chard.)

Slow Cooked Beans

Legumes are incredibly healthy, cheap, and easy. If you use a slow cooker, there's no need to pre-soak your beans, but doing so will remove many of the sugars and enzymes that cause intestinal discomfort.

There are almost no "rules" to cooking beans. You just put them in the cooker, cover them with water, and throw in what you like — an onion, some spices. Every half hour or so, you'll want to stir the pot and perhaps add water, but in about 5 hours, your beans will be ready to eat. A perfect meal for any day of the year, but especially on cold winter nights.

The Lonely Lentil

For some reason people just do not think about eating lentils. Nothing could be easier! Rinse your lentils under cold water and boil for 30 minutes or less. Make sure they're fully cooked to avoid gastric distress.

Perfect Vegetables to Sauté

Although sautéing isn't right for all vegetables (see the chapter on preferred cooking methods), it's perfect for cabbage, which shouldn't be overcooked. Heat breaks down the healthy nutrients in cabbage including the glucosinolates. Lightly sauté your cabbage and keep it crisp for maximum benefit.

Use the same method for kale, which is actually even healthier cooked. Add chopped onions and drizzle with extra virgin olive oil for a satisfying and healthy warm dish.

Not in the mood for kale? How about mustard greens prepared the same way, but drizzled with sesame oil to bring out their pungent, slightly peppery taste.

Go with Kasha, Not Rice

Once you've sautéed your vegetables, serve them over kasha instead of rice. Boil 1 cup of kasha (toasted buckwheat) with 2 cups water or bone broth for 10 minutes. Allow the mixture to stand for 5 minutes and add freshly cooked onions or vegetables!

Grow Your Own Salad Sprouts

Use sunflower seeds in the shell from the "black oil sunflower" to grow your own salad sprouts. It's easy, fun, and very healthy. Place your seeds in a large open-mouthed jar about half full of water. Don't be surprised when they float to the top; that's normal.

Seal the jar and allow the seeds to soak for eight hours. When they have doubled in size and the sprout has begun to emerge, rinse the seeds again and return to the jar in fresh water.

Cover the jar and let it sit for 1-3 days in a cool room with no direct sunlight. Rinse them again and return them to the jar for an additional 1-2 days. When the leaves have formed a "V" shape, the sprouts are ready to eat.

Other Super Food Ideas

Don't be afraid to experiment with incorporating superfoods into your recipes. Pumpkin, for instance, can be substituted for all the wet ingredients in brownies. That's right, add one can of pumpkin to one box of brownie mix and bake as directed.

Pumpkin is good for you in any form, and if you happen to use fresh pumpkin, save the seeds for toasting. Just 15-20 minutes in a 160-170 F oven and you'll have a crunchy, satisfying snack.

Substitute coconut oil for butter in your baking. It's naturally sweet, but contains no fructose. Heat won't harm coconut's healthy properties in the slightest. You can also toast coconut flakes or chips, and mix fresh coconut with your cereal.

Chapter 10 - Relevant Websites

10 Uncommon "Superfoods" From the World of Ultra-Endurance
www.huffingtonpost.com/tim-ferriss/10-uncommon-superfoods-fr_b_3361978.html

31 Superfood Secrets for a Long and Healthy Life
www.health.com/health/gallery/0,,20610379,00.html

Avocado Nutrition Facts - Six Things About This Amazingly Healthy Superfood
www.naturalnews.com/034370_avocado_nutrition_facts_health.html

Crouching Garnish, Hidden Superfood: The Secret Life of Kale
articles.mercola.com/sites/articles/archive/2013/11/06/kale-benefits.aspx

Dr. Fuhrman. Smart Nutrition. Superior Health.
www.drfuhrman.com

Dr. McDougall's Health & Medical Center
www.drmcdougall.com

Eat Healthy America: 52 Superfoods
www.womansday.com/health-fitness/nutrition/eat-healthy-america-52-superfoods-25519

Get a Taste for Teff, the Ethiopian Superfood
www.theguardian.com/global-development/poverty-
matters/2014/jan/23/get-taste-for-teff-ethiopia-superfood

Nutrition Facts
www.nutritionfacts.org

Peruvian Superfoods: The Most Powerful Powders on the
Planet
www.huffingtonpost.com/manuel-villacorta/peru-
superfood_b_3890210.html

Quinoa Rides the "Superfoods" Wave
online.wsj.com/articles/quinoa-rides-the-superfoods-
gluten-free-waves-1404926555

Superfoods: Are Chia Seeds and Goji Berries Really Good
for You?
www.tclegraph.co.uk/foodanddrink/10335775/Superfoods-
are-chia-seeds-and-goji-berries-really-good-for-you.html

Afterword

Now that you've worked through the text of this book, perhaps you can appreciate the following statement more fully — it's impossible to arrive at a definitive list of "superfoods."

Whenever I discuss this topic, I try to stick with the point I made in the Foreword. In investigating "superfoods" most people are really just trying to find their way back to *real* food.

It is true that the fruits, vegetables, grains, and herbs I discuss here stand out for their nutrient density and strong antioxidant properties. But it was not so long ago when a diet rich in fruits and vegetables was the rule rather than the exception.

We are the victims of a food culture that has come to focus on fast, processed, "food-like" substance to the point that the chemical-laden fare is cheap and affordable, and the healthy, nutritious food is often priced beyond reason under the label "organic."

There are so many factors to be concerned about in regard to diet today — additives, chemical contamination, genetically modified components — that a simple, unadulterated "carrot" suddenly gets elevated to "super" status.

The more you begin to incorporate real food into your diet, the closer you will be to a host of important goals —

improved cardiovascular health, decreased risk of diabetes, protection against cancer, and — or course — weight loss.

I've listed almost 100 foods in this book that qualify for "super" status. You don't have to eat them all. You may not even be able to eat them all. But you can certainly eat some of them, and make other modifications in your diet from what you've learned here.

There is nothing revolutionary about the idea of food as medicine. Our society is, in my opinion, focusing too much on reacting to illness rather than preventing it. Adopting a diet rich in super foods isn't a radical idea, it's a practical one — an idea I hope I've been able to make more accessible to you.

Glossary

ACE inhibitors - Present in whey protein, they regulate blood pressure and support overall cardiovascular health.

acetylcholine - A major neurotransmitter required for healthy brain function and good memory.

acetylenics - A compound found in celery that has been shown to halt cancer cell growth.

allicin - The active ingredient in garlic, believed to enhance immune function and prevent cancer among other purported benefits.

alliin - An amino acid found in garlic that interacts with the enzyme allinase to produce allicin, the active ingredient touted for its healthy benefits including cancer prevention and improvement of the immune system.

alpha-lactalbumin - Found in whey protein and believed to fight disease while improving mood and memory.

alpha linoleic acid - An omega-3 fatty acid that aids in reducing inflammation.

amino acids - Molecules that, when linked together, form proteins.

anethole - The compound that gives fennel its licorice flavor and is believed to reduce inflammation and inhibit the growth of cancer.

anthocyanins - The pigment molecules seen in especially vibrant fruits and vegetables like blueberries, red cabbage, and cherries red. Improves vision, guards against macular degeneration, enhances brain function, and reduces inflammation.

anthraquinone - A compound found in noni fruit that stimulates collagen synthesis and helps to prevent wrinkles.

antimutagenic - Possessing the power to slow the rate of mutation.

antioxidants - Compounds in food that combat oxidation and oxidative stress created by the activity of free radicals. This activity is a negative factor in virtually all degenerative diseases.

arginine - An amino acid that protects the lining of the arterial walls, increasing their pliability and resistance to the formation of plaque, a process known as atherogenesis.

astaxanthin - A carotenoid that inhibits lipid peroxidation and helps in mending DNA breakdown products.

avenanthramides - Unique to oats, these polyphenol antioxidants are anti-inflammatory and heart healthy.

beta-carotene - In the body, this carotenoid converts to Vitamin A.

betacyanin - An antioxidant compound also responsible for giving beets their red color.

beta-lactoglobulin - A protein fraction in whey that helps to preserve muscle during exercise and to inhibit cancer cells.

beta-sitosterol - A plant compound that regulates blood cholesterol and is beneficial for prostate health.

boron - A mineral believed to be important for bone and joint health, especially in women.

bran - The main source of fiber and nutrients in whole grains.

bromelain - A proteolytic enzyme extracted from pineapple that breaks down amino acids, fights inflammation, prevents blood clotting, relieves indigestion, and improves nutrient digestion.

caffeic acid - A strong antioxidant and anti-inflammatory found in coffee and rosemary.

capric acid - A medium-chain triglyceride found in coconut that forms into monocaprin in the human body where it increases levels of good cholesterol.

capsaicin - The active ingredient in hot peppers that is both an anti-carcinogenic and a vasodilator with pain-relieving properties.

carvacrol - An anti-fungal, antibacterial, and anti-parasitic compound found in oregano and thyme.

catechins - A group of polyphenols in green tea and cinnamon that are powerful antioxidants.

chalcone polymers - Phytochemicals in cinnamon that increase glucose metabolism.

charantin - A compound present in bitter melon believed to have anti-diabetic properties.

chlorogenic acid - Found in sweet potatoes, apples, and coffee, this powerful antioxidant targets an especially destructive free radical called the superoxide anion radical.

chlorophyll - A natural blood purifier and the compound responsible for the green color of plants.

choline - A nutrient essential for healthy liver and brain function and for the breakdown of fats. Found in eggs.

chromium - A trace mineral that helps in the function of insulin in the body.

conjugated linoleic acid (CLA) - A member of the omega family of fatty acids that helps to reduce body fat while fighting cancer and heart disease.

cortisol - An adrenal hormone with anti-inflammatory properties also effective in the regulation of blood pressure.

C-reactive protein - A protein in the blood that is used as a measure of inflammation in the body.

curcumin - A curcuminoid antioxidant with anti-inflammatory and anti-tumor properties. Also effective in lowering cholesterol.

diallyl disulfide - A compound found in garlic that has been shown to inhibit leukemia cells in laboratory testing.

diallyl sulfide - A compound in onions found to increase production of cancer-fighting enzymes.

diosgenin - A phytochemical present in beans that inhibits the multiplication of cancer cells.

dithiolethiones - Phytochemicals found in cabbage that have anti-cancer properties.

dopamine - A neurotransmitter in the brain referred to as a natural "feel-good" compound.

ellagic acid - A phenolic found in cherries and red raspberries with anti-carcinogenic properties and the ability to inhibit tumor growth.

epigallocatechin gallate (EGCG) - The catechin in green tea thought to be responsible for the drink's anti-cancer effects.

eritadenine - The active cholesterol-lowering compound found in shiitake mushrooms.

fiber - The indigestible component of food responsible for lowering the risk of heart disease, diabetes, obesity, and cancer

flavonoids - More than 4,000 plant compounds that have antioxidant, anti-cancer, and anti-allergy properties.

flavanols - Flavonoids found especially in cocoa that inhibit the clogging of the arteries by limiting the action of cholesterol in the bloodstream.

free radicals - Destructive molecules whose action in the body damages cells and DNA.

fucoidan - An anti-cancer polysaccharide found in kombu and wakame seaweed.

gamma-linoleic acid - A beneficial omega-6 fatty acid found in hemp seed, primrose, and borage oils.

ganodermic acid - A component in reishi mushrooms that regulates blood pressure and enhances liver and adrenal function.

gingerdiones - The active antioxidant in ginger.

gingerol - The phytochemical in ginger that gives the roots its pungent taste.

glycemic load - The measure of a food's effect on blood sugar.

glycyrrhizin - The saponin that is the active ingredient in licorice and is responsible for all of the plant's beneficial qualities.

haemagglutinin - A substance that promotes the formation of clotting in red blood cells. Found in soybeans among other foods.

hesperidin - The dominant flavonoid in oranges, hesperidin is anti-inflammatory, anti-allergic, vasoprotective, and anti-carcinogenic.

husk - The outer layer of a kernel of grain, also called chaff.

inflammation - The body's response to perceived attack, a self-protection mechanism that results in redness and swelling; regarded as a critical component in nearly all degenerative diseases.

insoluble fiber - The part of food that is indigestible and moves through the intestines in bulk.

insulin - A fat-storing hormone that, in a chronic elevated state, contributes to diabetes, cardiovascular disease, and aging.

inulin - A soluble fiber that occurs naturally for the purpose of feeding beneficial bacteria in the gut and supporting overall gastrointestinal health.

isoflavones - Found in soy foods, isoflavones ease the symptoms of menopause.

isothiocyanates - Anti-carcinogenic phytonutrients that neutralize cancer cells and stimulate the release of other substances that help to combat them.

lauric acid - A fat found in coconut oil with antiviral and antimicrobial properties that supports proper immune function.

L-ergothioneine - An antioxidant in mushrooms with a powerful neutralizing effect on free radicals and the ability to increase enzymes with antioxidant activity.

lignans - Plant compounds that protect against cancers, especially those with a strong hormone sensitivity like breast, uterine, and prostate cancers.

limonene - A phytochemical in citrus fruit peels that enhances the synthesis of antioxidant enzymes and aids in detoxification.

limonin - A limonoid present in lemons that lowers cholesterol.

lutein - A carotenoid with natural antioxidant properties for eye and skin health.

luteolin - A flavonoid in artichokes that prevents the oxidation of LDL cholesterol.

lycopene - A carotenoid found in tomatoes that is associated with a lower risk for prostate cancer.

lysine - An amino acid in quinoa that is scarce in vegetables.

macrophages - White blood cells that function as part of the body's natural defense system to destroy invaders like fungi and bacteria.

magnesium - A mineral useful in lowering high blood pressure.

malic acid - A substance in vinegar that fights toxins in the body and inhibits the growth of unfriendly bacteria.

manganese - A trace mineral needed for growth, reproduction, wound healing, brain function; and the metabolism of sugars, insulin, and cholesterol

methylhydroxychalcone polymer - The active ingredient in cinnamon, which mimics the function of insulin in the body for the management of glucose levels.

molybdenum - A mineral found in red kidney beans that enhances enzymes.

monocaprin - A by-product of capric acid with antiviral effects, found in coconut oil among other sources.

monoterpenes - Plant compounds found in essential oils derived from numerous fruits, vegetables, and herbs that has anti-carcinogenic properties.

monounsaturated fats - Fats found in nuts and olive oil among other sources, also called omega-9s, associated with lower incidence of heart disease.

mucopolysaccharides - Unique amino sugars found in the tissues of all multicellular organisms that combine with proteins in the body. They play a role in the proper structure of cartilage, bone, and elastic tissue, help to modulate the viscosity of fluids in the body, and normalize the bio-exchange of nutrients, electrolytes, and oxygen between capillaries and cells.

myricetin - A common flavonoid believed to have anti-inflammatory, anti-tumor, and antioxidant properties.

myristicin - A volatile oil present in parsley that is believed to inhibit the growth of tumors.

nasunin - A powerful antioxidant anthocyanin found in eggplant.

neochlorogenic acid - A phytonutrient present in plums and prunes that is especially effective against the superoxide anion radical, a very destructive free radical.

neoxanthin - A carotenoid present in spinach that causes the self-destruction of prostate cancer cells.

nitric oxide - A compound in the body that eases blood flow by relaxing constricted blood vessels.

octacosanol - A compound found in wheat germ oil believed to enhance exercise performance.

oleic acid - An omega-9 fat found in high concentration in macadamia nut oil, olive oil, and other nuts. It increases the ability of cell membranes to incorporate omega-3 fatty acids.

omega-3 fats - There are three kinds of unsaturated omega-3 fats: ALA (alpha-linoleic acid), DHA (docosahexanoic acid), and EPA (eicosapentanoic acid). EPA and DHA are found primarily in fish, while ALA is derived from nuts and seeds. These fats are highly beneficial.

ORAC value - The acronym for "oxygen radical absorbance capacity," which judges the power and effectiveness of an antioxidant.

organosulfur compounds - Anti-carcinogenic compounds found in kale.

oryzanol - A cholesterol-lowering compound present in brown rice.

osteocalcin - A compound activated by Vitamin K that has an anchoring effect on calcium molecules in bone.

oxalate - A substance present in many leafy greens that inhibits the absorption of calcium. For this reason, people who have trouble with kidney stones must limit their intake of oxalates.

pantothenic acid - The stress relieving vitamin B5, found in peanuts.

papain - A class of proteolytic enzymes that aid in the breakdown of proteins. Improves digestion and relieves pain. Extracted from papaya.

p-coumaric acid - A polyphenol antioxidant with anti-cancer properties.

pectin - A specific form of fiber useful to relieve constipation, lower cholesterol, and regulate blood sugar. Present in apples and quince.

perillyl alcohol - A compound in cherries believed to inhibit the growth of tumors.

phase-2 enzymes - Anti-carcinogens that interrupt the action of free radicals.

phenethyl isothiocyanate - A compound found in cruciferous vegetables like broccoli that is believed to be an anti-carcinogen.

phenolic compounds - A class of antioxidants that are useful in neutralizing the action of free radicals in the body.

phenols - Potent antioxidants and anti-inflammatory agents found in plants. Also known as phenolic acids.

phloridzin - A phytochemical with antioxidant properties found in concentration in apples.

phosphatidylcholine - A phospholipid that has choline as a component. Present in eggs, it helps to prevent the accumulation of fat and cholesterol in the liver.

phthalides - Phytochemicals present in celery that serve to increase blood flow while reducing levels of stress-causing hormones.

phycocyanin - A pigment that has both antioxidant and anti-inflammatory properties that may also inhibit the formation of cancer colonies.

phytates - Substances present in grains and soy foods that block mineral absorption.

phytic acid - Phytochemical present in beans that protects cells from genetic damage that can lead to cancer.

phytoalexins - Chemicals produced by plants that defend against attack by pathogenic microorganisms.

phytoene - An antioxidant present in fruits and vegetables, including tomatoes believed to have strong disease-fighting properties.

phytoestrogens - Compounds found in plants that have the ability to mimic the action of estrogen in the body.

phytofluene - An antioxidant present in fruits and vegetables, including tomatoes believed to have strong disease-fighting properties.

phytonutrients - Nutrients derived from plant sources.

phytosterols - Chemicals found in plants that have health benefits including the ability to lower cholesterol. Also called "plant sterols."

plant sterols - Alternate term for phytosterols. Chemicals found in plants that have health benefits including the ability to lower cholesterol.

phytosterols plasmin - An enzyme present in the body that works to dissolve and break down fibrin, which aid in the prevention of blood clots.

polyacetylenes - Compounds in plants that help to protect against potential carcinogens.

polyphenols - Antioxidants including flavonoids, anthocyanins, and isoflavones that protect cells from oxidative stress and the development of cancer.

polysaccharide - Chains of sugar units used by plants and animals for the storage of carbohydrates.

polyunsaturated fats - A class of fatty acids including both the omega-3s and the omega-6s. Found in vegetable oils, nuts, and fish. Oils with polyunsaturated fats are liquid at room temperature but solid when chilled. Lower the risk of heart attack.

proanthocyanidins - Antioxidants from plant compounds that are more potent than Vitamins C and E in protecting against environmental stresses like pollutants and cigarette smoke. Also protect against degenerative diseases.

probiotics - Bacteria that delivers beneficial effects for the digestive system. Found in naturally fermented foods and yogurt.

protease inhibitor - A phytochemical present in beans that has been shown to retard the division of cancer cells.

pterostilbene - A powerful antioxidant that fights cancer and lowers cholesterol.

purines - A substance found in cauliflower and other vegetables that breaks down uric acid in the body.

quercetin - A flavonoid that is both a natural anti-inflammatory and a powerful anti-carcinogen.

resveratrol - A phytoalexin compound known for its anti-aging effects and the ability to reduce both cardiovascular disease and the risk of cancer. Found in grapes and blueberries.

rosmarinic acid - A phenolic acid that is present in oregano and rosemary that has antimutagenic and anti-carcinogenic properties.

rutin - A bioflavonoid that helps to protect blood vessels. Found in asparagus.

saponin - Components of vegetables and legumes that act as natural antibiotics and exhibit anti-carcinogenic properties.

saturated fats - Saturated fats are solid at room temperature. Some forms, like those present in coconut oil, are beneficial, but the saturated fats found in most fast and processed foods raise cholesterol.

selenium - An essential trace element found in foods like Brazil nuts and chickpeas that has a strong anti-cancer effect.

serotonin - A neurotransmitter that has a mood-elevating effect while lowering the body's cravings for sugar.

sesamin - Found in sesame seeds, this member of the lignan family inhibits the development of inflammatory compounds in the body.

sesaminol - A phenolic antioxidant created when sesame seeds are refined into oil.

sesamol - A powerful antioxidant present in sesame oil and toasted sesame seeds.

shogaols - An active antioxidant component in ginger with strong inflammatory properties.

silicon - An important nutrient for bone health.

silymarin - A compound found in plants like milk thistle and artichoke that helps to nourish and protect the liver.

sinigrin - A chemical that suppresses the development of precancerous cells; present in Brussels sprouts.

sodium alginate - A compound in brown algae believed to reduce the uptake of radioactive particles into bone.

soluble fiber - Fiber that breaks down as it passes though the digestive tract where it forms a gel that traps cholesterol-raising substances. Also helps to control blood sugar.

stearic acid - A fat present in dark chocolate that has a neutral effect on the body.

steroidal glycosides - A compound present in asparagus root that effects hormone production and influences the emotions.

sterols - Fats that provide the basic molecule for key hormones in the body.

substance P - The chemical responsible for the transmission of pain signals to the brain.

sulfides - Sulfur compounds found in onions believed to regulate blood pressure and lower lipids.

sulforaphane - A member of the isothiocyanate family found in broccoli and broccoli sprouts. Offers protection against prostate, gastric, skin, and breast cancers.

superoxide dismutase (SOD) - An important antioxidant enzyme present in cereal grasses.

tannins - The chemicals in red wine and tea responsible for the astringent taste of the beverage.

taraxasterol - A constituent of dandelion instrumental in balancing hormones.

tartaric acid - An acid in vinegar that fights toxins in the body and inhibits the growth of harmful bacteria.

theaflavin - An antioxidant present in black teas.

theanine - The substance present in green tea responsible for the release of dopamine, a neurotransmitter with a calming effect.

thearubigen - An antioxidant present in black teas.

thujone - A compound present in oil of sage that is effective against salmonella and candida.

thymol - An antiseptic present in oregano and thyme that has anti-fungal, antibacterial, and anti-parasitic properties.

tocopherols - A compound found in olives that is part of the Vitamin E family and carries similar beneficial effects on the skin and connective tissues.

tocotrienols - antioxidants and heart-healthy nutrients present in palm oil, part of the Vitamin E family.

trans fat - The only beneficial trans fat is conjugated linoleic acid. All other forms increase the risk of developing cardiovascular disease.

triglyceride - The blood fat that is a significant risk factor in the development of cardiovascular disease.

turmeric - A pungent spice with strong anti-inflammatory properties.

tyrosine - An amino acid found in oysters converted in the human brain to dopamine.

umbelliferous - A group of vegetables identified by the National Cancer Institute as having cancer-protective properties; includes parsnips and parsley.

zeaxanthin - A carotenoid that is important for good eye health.

zera-carotene - An antioxidant present in many fruits and vegetables, including tomatoes that is believed to have strong potential for fighting disease.

zingerone - The antioxidant that is the active ingredient in ginger. It has anti-inflammatory properties and may be useful in managing conditions like arthritis and fibromyalgia.

Index

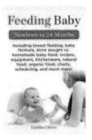

Feeding Baby
Cynthia Cherry
978-1941070000

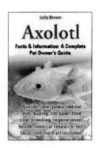

Axolotl
Lolly Brown
978-0989658430

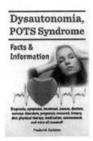

Dysautonomia, POTS
Syndrome
Frederick Earlstein
978-0989658485

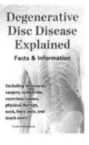

Degenerative Disc
Disease Explained
Frederick Earlstein
978-0989658485

Sinusitis, Hay Fever,
Allergic Rhinitis Explained
Frederick Earlstein
978-1941070024

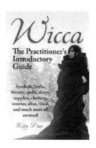

Wicca
Riley Star
978-1941070130

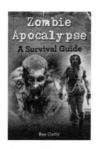

Zombie Apocalypse
Rex Cutty
978-1941070154

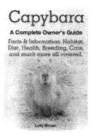

Capybara
Lolly Brown
978-1941070062

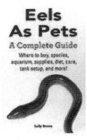

Eels As Pets
Lolly Brown
978-1941070167

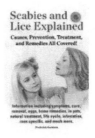

Scabies and Lice Explained
Frederick Earlstein
978-1941070017

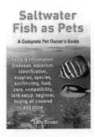

Saltwater Fish As Pets
Lolly Brown
978-0989658461

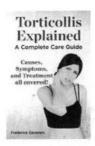

Torticollis Explained
Frederick Earlstein
978-1941070055

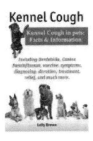

Kennel Cough
Lolly Brown
978-0989658409

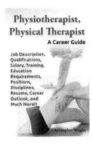

Physiotherapist, Physical
Therapist
Christopher Wright
978-0989658492

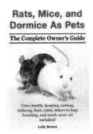

Rats, Mice, and Dormice
As Pets
Lolly Brown
978-1941070079

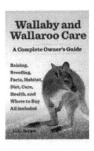

Wallaby and Wallaroo Care
Lolly Brown
978-1941070031

Printed in Great Britain
by Amazon